Say G...

Remember the freedom and flexibility you had *before* knee pain slowed you down? Now you can put the brakes on joint damage, heal the problem at the source, and free yourself from debilitating knee pain. Whatever the cause, this essential guide is the best first step to understanding the problem, choosing a doctor, and determining your treatment. Get ready to say hello to a whole new activity level and confidence of movement—and say goodbye to knee pain!

Also coauthored by Marian Betancourt—acclaim for

Say Goodbye to Back Pain

"An invaluable resource for understanding, diagnosing, and treating back pain."

> —Isadore Rosenfeld, M.D., *New York Times* bestselling author of *Dr. Isadore Rosenfeld's 2005 Breakthrough Health*

"Useful and informative. . . . Easy to understand yet comprehensive. . . . A great help for anyone who wants to have their back problems correctly diagnosed and treated."

> —Mathew H. M. Lee, M.D., Chairman, Rusk Institute of Rehabilitation Medicine

"A must read . . . for patients, doctors, and anyone dealing with back pain."

> —Harold F. "Pete" Garris, President, Matrix Medical Marketing

Say Goodbye to Knee Pain
is also available as an eBook.

Also by Marian Betancourt

Say Goodbye to Back Pain
  (with Emile Hiesiger, M.D.)

*What's in the Air? The Complete Guide to
  Seasonal and Year-Round Airborne Allergies*
  (with Gillian Shepherd, M.D.)

Say
Goodbye
to Knee
Pain

Jo A. Hannafin, M.D., Ph.D.,
and **Marian Betancourt**

POCKET BOOKS
New York   London   Toronto   Sydney

Pocket Books
A Division of Simon & Schuster, Inc.
1230 Avenue of the Americas
New York, NY 10020

Copyright © 2007 by Jo A. Hannafin, M.D., Ph.D.,
and Marian Betancourt

First Pocket Books paperback edition December 2007

POCKET and colophon are registered trademarks of
Simon & Schuster, Inc.

For information about special discounts for bulk purchases,
please contact Simon & Schuster Special Sales at
1-800-456-6798 or business@simonandschuster.com

Cover design by James R. Perales; cover photo © Jupiter Images

Manufactured in the United States of America

10 9 8 7 6 5 4 3 2

ISBN-13: 978-1-4165-4059-5
ISBN-10:   1-4165-4059-8

For John, Andrew, Caitlin, and Connor.

J.H.

For Dan Quirke,

who said goodbye to knee pain.

M.B.

ACKNOWLEDGMENTS

With thanks to my patients, who teach me daily, to my mentors for sharing their knowledge and guidance, and to my colleagues.

—J.H.

Thanks and gratitude to Nancy Love of Nancy Love Literary Agency and to Mara Sorkin, our editor at Pocket Books.

—M.B.

DISCLAIMER

The ideas, procedures, and suggestions in this book are not intended as a substitute for the medical advice of your trained health professional. All matters regarding your health require medical supervision. Consult your physician before adopting the suggestions in this book, as well as about any condition that may require diagnosis or medical attention. The authors and publisher disclaim any liability arising directly or indirectly from the use of the book.

CONTENTS

INTRODUCTION

Knees are a major source of pain for millions of people. Because they carry your weight all of your life and allow you to move around, these complex joints—the largest in your body—are vulnerable to all sorts of problems. Many causes of knee pain are preventable or modifiable, so seek medical attention early. People are often afraid to seek an evaluation because they don't want surgery. It is estimated that about ten million people in the United States visit orthopedic surgeons each year because of knee problems, according to national health statistics. But it is important to recognize that many knee conditions can be treated with medication, exercise, and simple lifestyle changes.

While knee replacement is a great advance in combating knee pain, we've also made advances in less invasive treatments. We know now, for example, that exercise and weight management can relieve arthritis pain. We know that physical therapy before surgery can improve the outcome of knee surgery by strengthening the muscles that support the knee.

Medicine is an ever-changing science, and this certainly applies to orthopedic care. New technologies are being developed every year to help us diagnose and treat knee injuries. New medications appear monthly. Techniques such as arthroscopic and minimally invasive surgery are becoming the norm. Hospital stays are shortening, and more and more testing and care are being rendered in the outpatient setting. The application of arthroscopy to assist in the diagnosis and surgical treatment of joint injury and disease has opened new horizons in therapy. The surgical management of degenerative joint disease such as arthritis has grown tremendously over the last twenty to thirty years, as has our ability to replace a diseased joint with a prosthetic device (total joint replacement). Surgeons are pursuing new treatment advances, including cartilage resurfacing and regeneration, that one day may prevent or delay the necessity for knee replacement.

This book will help you understand how your knees work, what can go wrong, and how to prevent or treat those conditions. You'll also learn how to find the right doctor to treat your knee pain, as well as what kinds of diagnostic tests may be required to get to the root of the problem. A chapter on physical therapy will help you understand why it is so important in most treatments for knee pain. And there are chapters on how to condition your body and make simple lifestyle changes that can help reduce knee pain.

PART I

THE BASICS

How Your Knees Work and Why They Hurt

Chapter 1

Anatomy of the Knee: The Body's Complex Joint

Jonathan is a young techie who knows all the parts of a computer, flat-screen television, mobile phone, and other miracles of the information age. The anatomy of these machines is easy for him to understand. He is well versed in gigabytes, Wi-Fi, motherboards, firewalls, Bluetooth, and RAM. However, when Jonathan's doctor told him that his persistent knee pain was caused by subluxation of his patella, he was clueless about such a simple yet important part of his own anatomy—the groove in which his kneecap glides. Perhaps his doctor should have compared it to the space bar on his computer keyboard, so he would understand why proper tracking in this groove is so important.

Jonathan is not alone. Many people know a lot more about the anatomy of technology than they do about their own bodies—the most precious "machine" they have. Your knee is your body's most complex joint, a crucial component of what makes you mobile, yet you might be hard-pressed to name parts of your knee beyond kneecap or tendon. There are other key components that you need to know about so you can maintain your knees in optimum health. Do you know how ligaments provide stability to your knees? Can you identify the two types of lubrication and cushioning that protect your knees? Would you be able to identify what is wrong if your knee pain is on the outside or inside of your knee, or in front? In order to prevent or treat any kind of knee pain, you need to know what makes your knees tick, literally and figuratively.

Your knees are built to carry your weight and hold up to a lifetime of walking, running, jumping, dancing, and all that you do in an upright or bent position. There is tremendous variability in the knee's response to activity, and this can be influenced by age, weight, gender, and genetics. Knees are vulnerable to damage from falls or sudden twisting motions, and are injured, on average, more frequently than other joints. Because your knee is such a complex joint, this chapter will help you understand the structure of your knees and what makes them prone to injury.

The motion of your knee is complex. It is somewhat like the hinge of a door, moving backward and forward, and like the elbow, it is capable of limited rotation. The knee is made of three bones held together by ligaments and works in coordination with muscles, tendons, cartilage, bursae, synovial fluid, and nerves. Your femur, the bone in your thigh, makes up the top part of the knee, and your tibia, the bone in your shin, the lower part. The third bone is the kneecap, also called the patella, which slides in a groove on the lower end of your thighbone. A fourth bone, the fibula, is a long narrow bone adjacent to your tibia that is connected by a

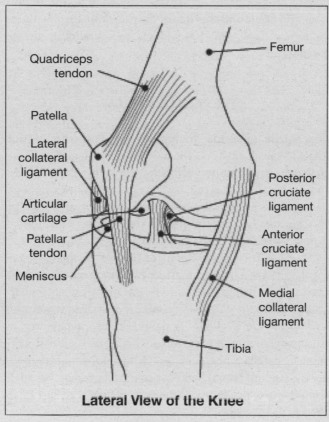

Lateral View of the Knee

FIGURE 1. This side view of the knee shows how the ligaments and tendons connect and support the femur, tibia, and patella. (*Courtesy of National Institute of Arthritis and Musculoskeletal and Skin Diseases, National Institutes of Health.*)

variety of soft tissue structures. The ends of the femur, tibia, and fibula and the back of the patella are lined with articular cartilage, which provides a smooth gliding surface for motion.

THE PATELLA: KNEECAP

Your patella is the small triangular bone in the front of your knee. The back of the patella is lined with articular cartilage so that it can glide smoothly in the groove located at the end of your femur. This is the trochlear groove. When you bend and straighten your knee, the patella moves up and down in this groove. Ideally, the patella remains centered in the groove as the knee bends and extends.

Your quadriceps muscles in the front of the thigh, via the quadriceps tendon, attach directly to the upper edge of the kneecap and help to keep it in its groove by exerting a balanced pull on the patella. Any imbalance in these structures, such as muscle weakness or tightness, has the potential to cause patellofemoral problems, including pain or maltracking. The patella is also stabilized by the retinaculum, which are medial and lateral bands of connective tissue that span from the patella to the distal femur, the part farthest from the patella (see below).

If the patella glides laterally toward the outside of the knee in this groove, this is known as patellofemoral maltracking. If the patella transiently comes out of the groove, this is a patellar subluxation and reflects that the patella is not tracking properly. When the patella is completely dislodged from the groove, this means that your kneecap is dislocated. There is an additional structure called the medial

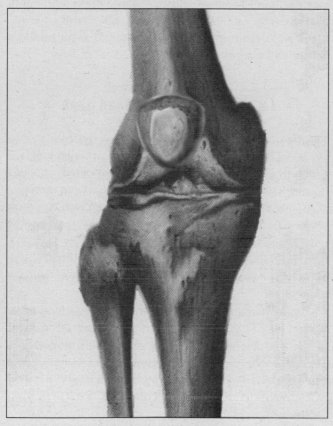

FIGURE 2. This frontal view of the knee with the muscles and tendons peeled back shows the bony alignment. (© *Olga Spiegel, 2007.*)

patellofemoral ligament (MPFL), a discrete thickening of the medial retinaculum. The strong band of connective tissue is important for patellar stability and can be torn in a patellar dislocation.

LIGAMENTS: THE FOUR STABILIZERS

The four ligaments that stabilize your knee are strong rope-like bands of collagen and elastin that link bone ends together to give mechanical stability to your knee, guide its normal motion, and help prevent abnormal motion. When ligaments are too lax, or loose, they don't hold your knee bones as firmly. Most laxity results from trauma and may require ligament reconstruction to restore stability. However, there are some people who are "loose jointed." They have many lax ligaments throughout the body, even without trauma.

The collateral ligaments run along the inner and outer sides of your knee. These are the medial collateral ligament (MCL) and lateral collateral ligament (LCL), respectively. The cruciate ligaments cross diagonally from the back of the femur to the front of the tibia (anterior cruciate ligament, or ACL) and from the front of the femur to the back of the tibia (posterior cruciate ligament, or PCL). The ACL and MCL are the most frequently injured ligaments, but damage can occur to any or all of them. These injuries can be serious and painful because ligaments are slow to heal.

If bones are pulled too far apart, ligament fibers overstretch, resulting in a sprain or tear. Ligament injuries are graded on a scale of 1 to 3, from a mild sprain to a complete tear. This is explained in chapter 7 about diagnosis. It's important to know these terms because your physician may use them when describing your condition. ACL injuries are common in contact sports, such as two players colliding on a football field, as well as noncontact situations, such as when you plant your foot and pivot suddenly to change direction. If you completely tear your ACL, you will know it immediately. You may feel intense pain, feel or hear a pop in your knee, and experience its giving way or instability. Your knee may swell within the first few hours following the injury even if you have applied ice to it. PCL tears are less common and occur when a force applied to the tibia drives the tibia backward. This can occur with a fall on a bent knee, a dashboard injury during a car accident, or contact with another athlete. The MCL is usually injured by a blow to the outside of the knee while the foot is planted. This force exerts pressure on the inside ligament, forcing the knee into a "knock-kneed" position. With this injury, you may feel a ripping sensation and the sense that your knee is buckling. The LCL is rarely injured by itself, but it can be injured in combination with an injury to the outer aspect of the knee.

Pain from sprained ligaments generally gets worse over the first twenty-four hours and is accompanied by knee

Top Sports for Contact ACL Injuries

Basketball
Football
Soccer
Lacrosse
Rugby

Top Sports for Noncontact ACL Injuries

Soccer
Basketball
Skiing
Lacrosse
Field hockey

swelling. The pain from a ligament injury usually gets worse when you walk or bend your knee.

TENDONS:
THE CONNECTION FROM MUSCLE TO BONE

Tendons connect muscle to bone and are among the strongest of any soft tissue in your body. They make it possible to use your muscles to bend and straighten your leg by changing the position of your knee joint. The quadriceps tendon connects the quadriceps muscle on the front of your thigh to the top of your kneecap. The patellar tendon connects your kneecap to the top of your tibia. The hamstring tendons connect the hamstring muscle on the back of your thigh to the tibia and fibula. The medial hamstring tendons attach to the tibia, and the lateral hamstring tendons attach to the fibula. So, essentially, the quadriceps tendon helps you straighten your knee, and the hamstring tendons help you bend it.

Like ligaments, the tendons are bands of tissue. However, they have more densely packed collagen than ligaments and can handle the high tensile loads required during activities such as rowing, running, cycling, jumping, and dancing. Most tendon injuries are caused by overuse, which can result in inflammation (tendinitis) or tendon degeneration (tendinosis), but some tendon injuries are caused by trauma. (See chapter 9 about treatment of tendinitis.)

ARTICULAR AND MENISCAL CARTILAGE: THE SHOCK ABSORBERS

There are two types of cartilage in your knee that are critically important to its normal function. They act as cushions, or shock absorbers, and help stabilize the knee joint.

Articular Cartilage

Articular cartilage is the smooth, shiny material that covers bone surfaces where they touch so they can glide easily: the ends of the femur, the trochlear groove, the top of the tibia, and the underside of the kneecap. Articular cartilage cannot regenerate, so when it is injured, it can be difficult to treat because time alone will not heal it. Instead, there are ways to resurface areas of traumatic cartilage loss, but these procedures result in formation of a fibrocartilage that is less desirable than articular cartilage. Loss of articular cartilage from aging or trauma results in osteoarthritis and pain. People with cartilage injury often ask if they have arthritis, which they view as a problem of the elderly. By definition, any damage to articular cartilage is a component of arthritis. It can be mild, moderate, or severe, and can affect a limited area of your articular cartilage or all of your cartilage surfaces.

Meniscal Cartilage (The Meniscus)

The cartilage known as the meniscus is made of two C-shaped, padlike structures of fibro-elastic cartilage that separate the surfaces of the femur and tibia. There is a meniscus on the medial and lateral sides of the knee joint.

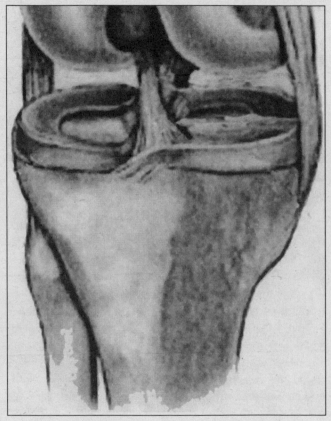

FIGURE 3. This close-up of the top of the tibia shows
how the meniscus acts as a cushion between it and the
femur. The menisci are two C-shaped pads, one on
the inner side of the knee and one on the outer side.
(© *Olga Spiegel, 2007.*)

Menisci is the plural for the two crescents that are found in each knee. They have a firm, springy structure and are made of collagen fibers interwoven with a gel-like material (proteoglycans) that, unlike the articular cartilage, *can* heal in specific regions.

Tears to the meniscus, commonly known as "torn cartilage," are a common cause of knee pain in people of all ages. Meniscus tears can cause swelling, stiffness, pain, limitation of motion, and mechanical symptoms such as catching or locking, where the knee feels like it is stuck in an unnatural position. In people under the age of thirty, torn cartilage is generally caused by trauma and related to an event such as a twisting injury. With increasing age, the meniscus begins to degenerate, becoming less springy and more fragile, so a tear can occur with something as simple as bending down to pick up something or playing a routine game of golf or tennis.

You may not notice small tears to the meniscus, but larger tears will usually cause pain and mild to moderate swelling. A displaced flap of torn meniscal cartilage can interfere with knee movement and can cause the knee to lock. Locking can also be caused by a piece of articular cartilage that has broken off and is floating in the joint cavity. This is known as a "loose body." You may not even notice it is a problem until it interferes with knee movement, like a pencil caught in a door. Locking from a meniscal or flap tear generally causes recurrent symptoms at the same site, while locking from a loose body can occur at different sites or in different knee positions as the fragment floats in the knee.

Cartilage loss—both articular and meniscal—can also be caused by inflammatory conditions such as rheumatoid arthritis and psoriatic arthritis. It is uncommon, but sometimes people are born with a discoid meniscus—that is, a circular pad rather than a crescent-shaped pad, which can predispose a person to meniscus injury (see chapter 4).

SYNOVIUM: THE SOURCE OF LUBRICANT

The synovium is a thin membrane that lines the knee joint and creates synovial fluid. Think of synovial fluid—an excellent natural lubricant—as motor oil for your knee. Just as motor oil keeps a car's gears from grinding against each other, so the synovial fluid keeps the parts of your knees well lubricated. There is a small amount of synovial fluid produced in a normal joint to provide lubrication for the articular cartilage and meniscus. However, with knee infections and inflammatory conditions such as rheumatoid or psoriatic arthritis, the concentration and type of cells in the synovial fluid is markedly increased. This causes changes in the consistency of the synovial fluid, and reduces its effectiveness as a natural lubricant because these inflammatory cells can produce enzymes that destroy articular cartilage and result in decreased motion.

BURSAE: THE GLIDERS

A bursa is a thin, fluid-filled sac formed by two layers of synovial tissue. There are many of these sacs (bursae) strategically located around your knee to facilitate gliding of soft tissue structures over underlying bone. In the knee, there are three main bursae: the prepatellar bursa, located between the skin and the kneecap; the pes anserine bursa that sits between the medial hamstrings and the tibia; and the iliotibial bursa that lies between the iliotibial band and the lateral femur.

Normally, a bursa has minimal fluid in it, but if it becomes irritated it can fill with fluid and become large and swollen, like a blister. Bursae can be seen on examination only when they are inflamed as a result of injury or disease. This inflammation is called bursitis. A direct blow or even bumping your knee can cause prepatellar bursitis. You can also develop bursitis if you spend lots of time kneeling.

Bursitis causes pain in different parts of the knee, depending on which bursae are affected. Pain may be on the inside of the knee at the tibia (pes bursitis), outside of the knee at the femur (ITB bursitis), or in the front of the knee between the patella and the skin (prepatellar bursitis). Warmth, swelling, and occasionally redness can develop, and you will feel aching or stiffness when you walk. If the prepatellar bursa is inflamed, you will have considerable pain when you kneel, because kneeling increases pressure against the patella. (See chapter 9 about treating bursitis.)

OTHER KNEE ANATOMY TO KNOW ABOUT

There are a few more parts of the knee you may want to know about.

Iliotibial Band

The iliotibial band (ITB) is a long, fibrous structure extending from the outside top of the femur to the outside top of the tibia. It helps rotate the hip and move the lower leg.

When your ITB is too tight it can rub against the femur, causing a dull ache or a sharp, burning pain. It also often results in inflammation, with repetitive bending and straightening of the knee.

The Retinaculum

The medial and lateral retinaculum are strong bands of connective tissue that help to stabilize the patella and hold your kneecap in place. A well-balanced retinaculum is important to the function of the patellofemoral joint. If the retinaculum is too tight, it may cause patellofemoral pain. If it is too loose, it may contribute to patellar instability.

Muscles: The Quadriceps and Hamstrings

The quadriceps is composed of four muscles that help to control the position of your kneecap and provide stability when you bend your knee: the vastus medialis (inner), vastus lateralis (lateral), vastus intermedius, and rectus femoris (central). The vastus medialis obliquus (VMO), which makes up a portion of the vastus medialis, helps to maintain the proper tracking of the patella in the trochlear groove.

The hamstrings run along the back of your thigh, and connect your pelvis and femur to the tibia and the fibula. The lateral hamstring is the biceps femoris, and the medial hamstring is composed of the semimembranosus and semitendinosus muscles. The gastrocnemius is the superficial calf muscle that provides the contour of the calf. The tendons of the medial and lateral heads of the gastrocnemius cross the knee joint and attach to the posterior distal femur.

KEY POINTS

- Knees are the largest and most complex joints in your body.
- Ligaments are attached to the large upper and lower leg bones to provide stability.
- Tendons are attached to the muscles in the front and back of the thigh to allow you to move your legs and control the kneecap.
- The patella—kneecap—moves up and down in the front of your knee in the trochlear groove.
- Articular and meniscal cartilage cushion your knees, but once articular cartilage wears out, it cannot regenerate.
- Synovial fluid coats all the parts of your knee to provide lubrication.
- Bursae are small fluid-filled sacs that help to ease movement in your knee.
- Other muscles and connective tissues help stabilize and support your knee's range of motion.

Chapter 2

Common Risk Factors
for Knee Pain

Whether you are an athlete or a couch potato, you are at risk for knee pain. You may be at higher risk for traumatic knee problems if you are an athlete, but the risk of traumatic knee pain also increases if you are overweight, if you lack strength and flexibility, or if you come from a family with a history of knee problems. Women are also more vulnerable than men to certain types of knee pain, and not all knee pain comes late in life. There are particular risks at various life stages, from childhood to old age, as you will learn in the following chapters.

BEING OVERWEIGHT

Anna, sixty-two, tripped and fell while walking with her five-year-old granddaughter one day. The child had suddenly cut in front of her, and Anna, trying to avoid falling over her granddaughter, lost her balance and fell.

She fractured her kneecap in three places even though the fall was not very forceful. However, Anna was sixty pounds overweight, a factor that added force to the fall. Anna needed open surgery to repair her kneecap and then had to use a walker and eventually a cane to get around. This initially made her feel like an invalid, but she soldiered through months of physical therapy to get back to normal. Today she is back to walking normally, but the injury to the cartilage in her knee makes Anna a candidate for developing posttraumatic arthritis.

Being overweight is one of the leading risk factors for knee pain. Even ten pounds over your ideal weight can cause knee pain by increasing the stress on your knees during ordinary activities such as walking or going up and down a flight of stairs. For example, when you walk down stairs, your kneecap experiences a force equal to two to three and a half times your body weight. Thus, 50 pounds of excess weight can place an additional 150 pounds of pressure on your kneecaps every time you walk down a step. This added burden to your knees can accelerate the breakdown of cartilage and put you at increased risk of developing osteoarthritis. Knee pain is also becoming a problem for the increasing number of children who are overweight.

PREVIOUS INJURY

If you have dislocated your kneecap, sprained a ligament, or torn your meniscus, you may be more likely to have knee pain in the future from a recurring injury. Frank, a firefighter, injured his knees repeatedly while playing football in high school and college, and also on the job. He became a candidate for knee replacement at age fifty because medical treatment such as medication, physical therapy, and arthroscopic debridement (smoothing away rough and damaged cartilage) were no longer effective in managing his pain. It is well known that injury to articular cartilage contributes to the development of posttraumatic arthritis. Loss of a significant portion of the meniscus can result in early osteoarthritis.

Cutting-and-pivoting sports such as Alpine skiing, basketball, soccer, and football put significant stress on your knees. The sharp twists and turns, falls, or collisions increase the potential for knee damage. In fact, most contact sports affect knees. It is important to be physically prepared for your sport with appropriate strength and endurance training to decrease the risk of injury. This does not mean you should stop playing sports, but you need to rethink the sports that you participate in if you have already sustained multiple knee injuries.

OVERUSE

Overuse injuries can happen to both athletes and people who engage in repetitive everyday behaviors that put strain on their knees.

Cheryl, thirty-four, was a single mom with a full-time administrative job at a hospital. Since her high school days, she always loved to run because it gave her a feeling of freedom. After running short distances daily be-

came a cherished routine, Cheryl decided to compete in her city's marathon. While she had a sensible routine for conditioning herself year-round for shorter distances, Cheryl went overboard while training for the marathon and overworked her knees with poorly designed practices, adding too many additional miles and pushing herself on more grueling terrain, such as steep hills. She began developing pain on the outside of her knees shortly after beginning her daily run. At first, she tried to slow down a bit, but the pain persisted and began bothering her even after she stopped running. Finally, after getting a thorough checkup, she discovered that she had iliotibial band syndrome, a common overuse injury in runners. A well-designed stretching program, physical therapy, and education in marathon training was the solution to her painful knees, and helped her complete the marathon.

Jack, forty-one, owned a small flooring and carpet-laying business and spent a good deal of his time on his knees. He was a strong, healthy man who didn't always remember to use protective knee pads when he was in a hurry. Given the normal pressures of a small contracting business, Jack sometimes had to spend many hours on his knees in order to get a job finished on time. Eventually the pain and swelling in his knees were keeping him from doing his work, so he went to the doctor and discovered he had developed severe prepatellar bursitis.

As you age, your kneecap is a common source of knee pain from repetitive bending, as in pedaling a bike or kneeling. The muscles around the knee can become less flexible and can result in overload of the knee. This may cause an inflammatory response that damages cartilage or the tendons that attach muscle to the knee. An inflammatory response is your immune system sending more blood (resulting in redness and warmth) and other body chemicals (resulting in swelling) to the site of a problem.

Your body needs time to recover, or the cycle of inflammation and microdamage continues and increases your risk of injury. It is not repeated motion itself that is to blame, but, rather, the lack of adequate recovery time. The tissue in and around the knee can't heal if you subject your knee to overload. Eventually the pain will become chronic and can lead to arthritis. This is why strength-training guidelines always advise against working the same muscle group on consecutive days.

LACK OF MUSCLE FLEXIBILITY OR STRENGTH

John, forty-five, drives a bus in a busy section of a major city. One day, while assisting a passenger in a wheelchair, John squatted down to adjust the straps that hold the chair in place. He felt a sudden, excruciating pain in his knee and was forced to ask other passengers to help him stand up. He rubbed his knee and limped back to the driver's seat but was in pain for the rest of the day. Later, his doctor told John he had torn his meniscus and would be out of work for several days. At the end of his work day, John usually went home and stretched out on the couch to relax. His doctor encouraged him to begin an early morning exercise and conditioning program, before he went to work, so he wouldn't feel too tired to do it at the end of the day. Had his muscles been stronger, John might not have injured himself when he bent to adjust the wheelchair.

Lack of flexibility and strength are among the leading causes of knee injuries and acute pain. When your muscles are weak, they offer less support for your knee because they don't absorb enough of the stress exerted on your knee joints. In women, patellar pain—pain in front of the knee—is often caused by a lack of strength in the quadriceps and hip musculature. In general, with the onset of hormonal changes, middle-aged and older women are more likely to lack muscle strength or endurance, while men are more likely to lack muscle flexibility. Both genders can have a difficult time maintaining or increasing muscle mass. (See chapter 18 about conditioning.)

KEY POINTS

- Being overweight is a significant risk factor for knee pain and development of osteoarthritis.
- Failure to keep leg muscles flexible and strong is a risk factor for knee pain.
- Cutting-and-pivoting sports such as Alpine skiing, football, soccer, volleyball, and basketball can result in injury and early knee pain.
- Overuse injuries from repetitive strain on the knee are a risk factor for knee pain.

SEVEN WAYS TO REDUCE YOUR
RISK FOR KNEE PAIN

1. Maintain a healthy weight to minimize additional pressure on your knees.
2. If you have suffered knee injuries in the past, be more vigilant about conditioning exercises or physical therapy to strengthen your knees and decrease your risk for further injury and pain.
3. Make stretching and strengthening your hip, thigh, and calf muscles a part of your normal routine.
4. Give your body time to rest between bouts of repetitive activity such as running, cycling, or kneeling.
5. Wear protective knee pads when kneeling for any length of time.
6. Cross-train to maintain fitness; alternate cardiovascular and strength training; vary your aerobic exercise program to prevent overuse injury.
7. If you participate in cutting-and-pivoting sports that put you at risk for ACL injury, consider enrolling in an injury prevention program.

Chapter 3

The Differences in Men's and Women's Knees

More women than men suffer from knee pain. According to 2006 statistics from the Centers for Disease Control and Prevention, 22 percent of women aged forty-five to fifty-four have knee pain, while only 19 percent of men in the same age group report knee pain. Also, the type and frequency of knee pain suffered differs according to gender. Men are statistically more likely to suffer from gout, while women are more likely to develop osteoarthritis. Boys more frequently have pain from Osgood-Schlatter disease, which affects the growth plate (specialized cells on the growing end of the bone) attachment of the patellar tendon, while girls have more problems and pain related to their patellofemoral joints. Young men are more likely to suffer traumatic injuries to the knee, while female athletes are more likely than male athletes to sustain a noncontact injury to their anterior cruciate ligament (ACL).

THE FEMALE ATHLETE'S ACHILLES HEEL
IS ACTUALLY THE KNEE

Throughout history, women were discouraged from playing competitive sports. In Victorian times, for example, women were so encumbered by corsets, petticoats, and layers of fabric that it's lucky they could move at all. The male establishment claimed that women were too frail, too weak, or would get "the vapors" if they participated in sports. Yet for most of medical history, women were treated by the same establishment as if they were smaller versions of men. Today we know that this is not true. Men and women have significant differences in disease presentation, response to medications, body chemistry, and gross anatomy—including the knees.

While both men and women can develop knee pain, certain types of problems are more common in one gender than the other. The noncontact injury to the ACL is one example of a recognized gender difference in knee injury. Noncontact ACL injury is three to four times more common in women than in men participating in comparable sports such as basketball, soccer, and volleyball. The reason for this gender difference remains unclear but likely results from many causes. Several theories have been proposed, including anatomic alignment (the difference in the angle of a woman's hip, knee, and ankle), hormonal action, and neuromuscular training and balance.

According to the National Collegiate Athletic Association (NCAA), women playing soccer and basketball suffer three to five times more ACL injuries than men. Others have reported that the injury is five to eight times more common in women. The American Orthopaedic Society for Sports Medicine estimates that ten thousand women experience debilitating knee injuries a year at the college level. At the high school level, this statistic rises to twenty thousand. Pivoting and jumping are moves that put the knee at risk and are common in soccer, basketball, and volleyball.

Women, in general, have less muscle mass than men, which affects knee function. Differences in muscle mass, muscle reaction time, and muscle firing patterns are different in men and women and may predispose women to injury. Women more often have a narrow intercondylar notch (the "home" of the ACL), which may increase the risk of noncontact ACL injury in specific women.

It has been proposed that monthly hormonal fluctuations play a role in the increased incidence of noncontact ACL injury in women. This may occur via alteration in the strength or flexibility of women's ligaments or may affect neuromuscular parameters such as jumping, landing, balance, proprioception (body position in space), or reaction times. It is not yet clear how hormones play a role in ACL injury, but there is extensive ongoing research designed to ask and answer some of these questions. Women also tend to run, jump, and land in a more upright position and use their hip, quadriceps, and hamstring muscles differently than men. You can't change your body structure, but studies show that women can significantly reduce their risk of ACL injury by strengthening the muscles surrounding the knee and improving movement patterns involved in landing, pivoting, or stopping quickly.

Extensive research continues at medical and sports centers around the country to determine why females sustain this type of injury at increased rates and to develop injury-prevention programs. (For more information about injury-prevention programs, see the resources in the appendix.)

VENUS AND MARS THROUGH THE AGES

The causes of knee pain in men and women differ according to age. For example, in adolescent and young adult men, traumatic injury to the knee (fractures, meniscus tears, ligament injury) is most common. In the same age group of females, the most common condition is patellofemoral pain, followed by sports-related traumatic knee injury. Young adult women also suffer more knee pain from rheumatoid arthritis and other autoimmune diseases than men.

In the middle-aged population, degenerative meniscal tears and early osteoarthritis are common in both men and women, and there is a moderate subpopulation of women with patellofemoral arthritis—often the same women who have had the pain since adolescence. While women are more vulnerable to arthritis, men get gout more often, a type of inflammatory arthritis caused by uric acid crystals building up in the knee joint.

In the mature population, osteoarthritis is more common in women than men. Women are also heavier than they used to be, and obesity contributes to knee pain. A study by the Centers for Disease Control and Prevention reported in 2006 that 67 percent of American women ages forty-five to fifty-four are overweight, compared to 49 percent in 1960. There is recent scientific evidence to suggest that the biologic behavior of articular cartilage in women is different than in men and may predispose them to early cartilage degeneration that is unrelated to their body weight.

REPLACING HIS AND HERS

The designs of knee prostheses vary from company to company, but until recently, the role of gender in the design of knee replacements had not been considered. Women and men received the same prostheses in different sizes. However, the differences in the bony anatomy of the male and female knees have been considered in the newer gender-specific prosthesis designs. This may be good news, as women currently comprise the majority of people getting knee replacements. Long-term outcome studies are needed before we can determine whether or not the gender-specific prosthesis will make a substantial difference for women. We do know that women have an increased incidence of knee stiffness following total knee replacement. The cause of this difference is not yet known.

There are also known gender differences in the utilization of medical services. It has long been noted that men are more reluctant than women to be evaluated by a doctor when something is wrong. This has been studied with regard to medical issues but not to knee problems specifically. The general population is becoming more aware of health issues, and men seem more willing to seek medical help.

KEY POINTS

- More middle-aged women than men report knee pain.
- Women generally have a narrower notch where the anterior cruciate ligament is attached to the femur.

- Women are three to four times more vulnerable to ACL injury than men.
- Women tend to run, jump, and land in a more upright position and use their hip, quadriceps, and hamstring muscles differently than men.
- Adolescent boys are more prone to traumatic knee injury, while girls are more likely to develop pain in the front of the knee (patellofemoral pain).
- Rheumatoid arthritis and other autoimmune diseases are more common in women than in men.
- In older adults, osteoarthritis is more common in women than in men.
- Knee replacement surgery is beginning to adapt to the physical differences between genders in the structure of the knee.

Chapter 4

Knee Pain in Childhood and Adolescence

Two simultaneous and seemingly contradictory developments in our culture are setting the stage for enormous increases in knee pain in children: increased childhood obesity and the increasing number of children playing competitive contact sports. This seems quite a conundrum, since participation in aerobic sports at an early age will help combat obesity. While obesity will put pressure on the knees at an earlier age, a child's developing bones and joints are also vulnerable to sports injury, particularly with participation in contact sports. Parents, coaches, and physicians need to find the correct balance between inactivity, joint overload, and traumatic injury. You will find more information about traumatic injuries in the young adults section of the next chapter.

Children's bodies don't grow in perfect synchronicity. Different parts of the body develop at different times and at their own pace. Growing children sometimes appear gangly or "coltish," seeming to be all arms and legs. The same thing occurs inside the body. Bones can grow in length at a faster rate than the ability of the soft tissues to adapt. This can result in pain around the knee during rapid growth spurts. In addition, young children's muscles may not be strong enough to protect the knee until the onset of puberty, when muscle development increases dramatically.

The growing bones of children are different from the bones of older adolescents and adults. Bones grow by adding new bone at the physis, or growth plate. The physis is an area of specialized cartilage present near the end of long bones, where longitudinal growth of bone occurs until skeletal maturity. Repetitive trauma to the immature growth plate—say, from jumping in gymnastics—or acute trauma, such as a fracture, has the potential to seriously injure the developing physis. This can result in growth arrest or asymmetric growth of the tibia or femur. Because these injuries can affect the growth of the bone, they should be evaluated and treated by a pediatric orthopedist.

Trauma from sports injuries is another leading cause of knee pain in children and adolescents because they are playing much more competitively than in the past. They share such injuries with young adults, and this is covered in depth in the next chapter about young adults.

There are other common causes of knee pain in growing children that can limit activity, such as the following conditions:

OSGOOD-SCHLATTER DISEASE

Darren, eleven, is a forward on his school's soccer team. The training regimen includes quite a bit of running,

kicking, and jumping, which caused Darren to develop
pain in the front of his left knee and some swelling at the
top of his shin, where his patellar tendon connects to the
tibia. Darren didn't want to stop playing, so he didn't
tell anyone about his pain until one day he confided in
his sister, who immediately reported it to his parents.
Darren's parents knew how important the game was to
their son, so they took him to his pediatrician for evalu-
ation before any decisions were made. The doctor diag-
nosed Osgood-Schlatter disease and explained how
Darren's running and lack of flexibility were causing the
pain. X-rays were taken, and a separation in the growth
plate was seen. The physician explained to Darren and
his parents about modifying his training and competi-
tion schedule. Darren was unable to play for several
weeks until his pain resolved and then slowly increased
his activity and returned to play.

Osgood-Schlatter disease (also called tibial tubercle apophysitis) is an overuse injury that affects athletic young people during the years when their bones are growing rapidly—usually ages ten to fifteen for boys, and eight to thirteen for girls—and is especially common in children who engage in sports year-round. It was first identified in 1903 and is more common in boys than in girls. However, the number of preadolescent girls participating in intensive sports has increased in recent years, and as a result, Osgood-Schlatter disease seems to be increasing in adolescent girls.

Osgood-Schlatter disease develops from repeated trac-
tion, or tugging, of the patellar tendon on the tibial apophysis (growth plate) at the top of the tibia—the front of the
shin. It is a form of continuous microtrauma and occurs

during activities that involve bending, running, and jumping, when the pull of the quadriceps muscle puts tension on the patellar tendon. The tendon attachment eventually begins to pull away from the tibia, resulting in a small, visible bump just below the kneecap that is painful to touch. When severe, the tendon may partially separate from the tibia and may take a fragment of bone along with it. Rarely, the tendon and a small fragment of bone completely separate from the tibia. To ensure that this does not happen, it is important for a young person to be evaluated by a doctor. Swelling may cause the patellar tendon to thicken. The location of the pain and swelling is at the top of the shin, just below the knee joint, and usually worsens with activity and is relieved by rest.

The symptoms generally resolve when a child stops growing because of closure of the tibial growth plate. In some susceptible teenagers, symptoms may last two to three years, but most cases of Osgood-Schlatter disease will completely resolve with completion of the growth spurt at about fourteen for girls and sixteen for boys. (See chapter 9 about diagnosis and treatment.)

PATELLAR SUBLUXATION AND DISLOCATION

Patellar subluxation and dislocation are forms of patella instability often present in adolescents when they increase their physical activity. A patellar subluxation occurs when your patella slides laterally out of position in its groove but doesn't completely dislocate. A patellar dislocation means that it *has* come out of the groove—often locking over the side of your knee. Both conditions can be caused by trauma, but they can also happen to you if you are loose jointed, meaning that your ligaments are more lax and don't support your knee as well as they should. A well-balanced patella glides up and down in the trochlear groove on the end of your femur as the knee bends and strengthens. Your kneecap is designed to fit in the center of this groove and slide evenly within it. When your kneecap is pulled toward the outside of your knee, it puts you at risk for pain around your kneecap or episodes of subluxation.

The kneecap can also sublux if the alignment of your thigh and shin is abnormal. An angle—called the Q angle—is created by the intersection of the long axis of the shafts of the femur and tibia. An increase in the Q angle is commonly seen in people with a knock-kneed, or valgus, alignment of the knee. There are also differences in the shape and depth of the trochlear groove. A shallow or flat trochlea increases your risk of patellar subluxation.

The quadriceps and hamstring muscles support your knee, and one of the quadriceps muscles, the vastus medialis oblique (VMO), on the inside of your knee, is important in stabilizing a loose patella. This muscle pulls your kneecap toward the middle of your joint and helps to maintain its position. If your VMO is not as well developed as other muscles around your knee, or if its muscle fibers are not adequately oriented to control the kneecap, then subluxation may result. Depending on the severity, this maltracking (the way the patella glides in the groove) may cause no symptoms, or it can result in anterior knee pain, subluxation, or dislocation. Most commonly, the abnormal tracking causes discomfort with activity and pain around the edges of the kneecap. If your patella subluxes, it is more likely to dislocate if you fall or injure your knee. However, if you have loose ligaments, a fall or trauma can cause the initial dislocation.

When your kneecap dislocates, the result is intense pain, swelling, and difficulty walking or straightening your knee. Patella dislocations resulting from trauma often require an emergency room visit to put the patella back into its normal position, while those caused by patellar laxity may move back spontaneously.

Once you have dislocated your kneecap, you are at increased risk of having it happen again. The good news is that you may not experience as much pain and swelling with subsequent episodes, but repeated dislocations can lead to chronic knee pain and damage to the underlying cartilage. Chronic subluxation will ultimately result in loss of cartilage in the patellofemoral joint, leading to early arthritis in this part of your knee. It is important to have an evaluation performed by a sports medicine physician or a pediatric orthopedic surgeon if you have had a patellar dislocation.

PATELLOFEMORAL PAIN AND CHONDROMALACIA OF THE PATELLA

Patellofemoral pain—pain in front of the knee and around the kneecap—is often seen in adolescent and young adult females. Such pain is a clinical diagnosis for localized pain in the area of the kneecap. Chondromalacia of the patella is a cause of patellofemoral pain that sometimes affects adolescents but is more common in adults. In this case, there is damage to the cartilage of the patella. Chondromalacia is a diagnosis that is made at the time of surgery or MRI evaluation and describes structural damage to the cartilage of the patellofemoral joint.

Either condition can result from too much pressure on the cartilage lining the deep surface of the patella. It can occur because of overuse, patellar instability, patellar mal-tracking, or overcompression of the patella. We tend to see patellofemoral pain in people who are "too loose" or "too tight." This is a bit of an oversimplification, but it helps in the initial assessment of someone with anterior knee pain. (See chapter 5 about this condition.)

OSTEOCHONDRITIS DISSECANS (OCD)

Osteochondritis dissecans is most common in adolescents and young adults who are active in sports. The cause of OCD of the knee is unclear, but it is related to loss of the blood supply to an area of bone and cartilage in the knee joint. (This can also occur in other joints, such as the elbow or ankle, but the knee is most common.) A fragment of bone with its overlying articular cartilage undergoes necrosis (bone death) and can begin to separate from the surrounding bone. The most common site is the inner back half of the medial femoral condyle. The affected bone and cartilage can separate, become mobile, and cause pain or catching. For example, this may happen to the elbow of a baseball pitcher from the repetitive strain. When it occurs in knees, it often presents in active athletic children and young adults. It is unclear if the activity helps to cause OCD, or if the activity results in symptoms that lead to the diagnosis.

Symptoms include a deep aching in the knee when walk-

ing, running, and playing sports. If the fragment is beginning to loosen, you may also feel as if your knee is giving way
and/or does not have full range of motion; perhaps you feel
a sticking sensation or like the knee is locking. You might
also hear a clicking sound when you do a deep knee bend.
Most people with OCD of the knee do not have a history of
trauma. (See chapter 8 about treatment.)

ILIOTIBIAL BAND (ITB) SYNDROME

Iliotibial band syndrome is an overuse injury that affects
teenagers, young adults, and more mature athletes, especially runners and cyclists. Pain is commonly present along
the ITB as it crosses over the end of the femur or at the attachment site of the ITB to the tibia on the outside of the
knee. This syndrome develops from an overly tight ITB that
is subjected to friction along the femur as the knee goes
through a repetitive arc of bending and straightening. A
small bursa, present between the ITB and the lateral side of
the femur, can also become inflamed in ITB syndrome. (See
chapter 9 about treatment.)

DISCOID MENISCUS

*Anthony is a seven-year-old whose parents noticed that
he was favoring one leg while walking. His mother also
began to notice a clicking noise when he bent down or
climbed a steep staircase. Though Anthony was not in
pain, he was unconsciously altering his walk because he
was self-conscious about the noise his knee was making.*

The boy's knee began to swell, and his parents took him to a pediatric orthopedist who discovered that Anthony had a discoid lateral meniscus, a benign developmental abnormality in which the meniscus is shaped like a disc rather than the normal C shape. This abnormality is most common in the lateral meniscus on the outer side of the knee, and it can cause a clicking sensation with or without pain.

Approximately 5 percent of the population are born with a discoid meniscus, and it is slightly more common in people of Asian descent. There are a number of variants of discoid meniscus. Some are unstable and move excessively, while others are well attached to the capsule of the knee joint. The discoid meniscus can tear and cause pain even in the absence of significant trauma. In some cases, the discoid meniscus must be surgically repaired or removed, while in others there may be no significant symptoms, and so the patient can simply be monitored.

JUVENILE RHEUMATOID ARTHRITIS (JRA)

Alice is a five-year-old who began to feel stiffness in her legs when she woke up in the morning. Sometimes she told her parents that her knees hurt, but because the pain and stiffness frequently seemed to subside once she got to kindergarten and when she was home later in the day, they thought perhaps she was reluctant to get up and go to school. After all, it was her first year. The condition persisted, and her parents thought that perhaps her bed wasn't comfortable, so they got her a new ortho-

pedic mattress. Because Alice began to complain about pain in multiple joints, her pediatrician referred her family to a pediatric rheumatologist, who diagnosed juvenile rheumatoid arthritis.

It is rare for children to develop the types of arthritis that affect adults, but juvenile rheumatoid arthritis (JRA) is the exception. Rheumatoid arthritis is a disease of the autoimmune system that can affect any—and sometimes all—the joints in the body, and occurs when the immune system attacks itself as if the body's own cells were a foreign invader. Doctors still don't know why the immune system goes awry in children with JRA, but it is suspected of being a two-step process. First, something in the child's genetic makeup suggests the tendency to develop JRA. Then an environmental factor, such as a virus, triggers the development of the disease.

Symptoms of JRA include joint inflammation, redness, swelling, soreness, and stiffness for more than six weeks, although some children with this disease do not complain of pain. The most common symptoms of JRA are persistent joint swelling, pain, and stiffness that typically are worse in the morning. Lymph nodes in the neck and other areas may swell, and in fewer than half the cases, internal organs may be affected. The disease may also interfere with growth in the affected limb. If the arthritis is more severe in one knee, for example, the growth of one leg may be slower or faster than the other, causing a leg length discrepancy.

There are three types of JRA:

Pauciarticular JRA, the most common type, affects fewer than four joints but usually the largest ones, so the knee is a common site. Approximately half of children with

JRA have this type. Girls under age eight are most likely to develop it. Because of the particular antibodies formed in the body, children with this disease also tend to develop eye disease. Some children with this type of JRA outgrow it by adulthood, although eye problems may recur later in life.

Polyarticular JRA affects about 30 percent of children and involves five or more joints, most commonly the smaller joints in the hands and feet. This type is often symmetrical, affecting the same point on both sides of the body. This is a more severe form of JRA, and affected children have elevated rheumatoid factor in their blood. It is similar to the adult version of rheumatoid arthritis.

Systemic JRA affects about 20 percent of cases and is sometimes called Still's disease. This form is characterized by fever and a skin rash in addition to joint symptoms. It may affect internal organs such as the heart, liver, spleen, and lymph nodes. It is the most severe of the three types of JRA.

PSORIATIC ARTHRITIS

Psoriatic arthritis occurs among people with the chronic skin condition psoriasis. While it is most common in adults, it does affect children as well. (See chapter 10 about treatment of this form of arthritis.)

SEPTIC ARTHRITIS

Septic arthritis, also called bacterial or infectious arthritis, is caused by an infection in the knee joint that results in pain, swelling, and a fever. Septic arthritis can occur at any age, but in children it is most common under the age of three. In an infant, septic arthritis may cause fever and immobility of the affected leg, or crying when the infected joint is moved. An older child or teenager·will have pain and swelling in the affected joint. The presence and degree of fever depend on the virulence of the bacteria.

The knee and hip are the most common sites for septic arthritis. Symptoms usually occur rapidly once the bacteria spread from a source of infection through the bloodstream to a joint, such as the knee. Sometimes an injury or surgical procedure can result in the infection. The most common type of infection following surgery is a staph infection from skin bacteria such as Staphylococcus aureus or Staphylococcus epidermidis. Other risk factors include a chronic illness that requires medications to suppress the immune system. Children with septic arthritis are more likely than adults to be infected with Group B streptococcus and Haemophilus influenza.

After age three, septic arthritis is less common. However, it is seen again in adolescents and young adults with gonorrhea. An adolescent or young adult may develop septic arthritis because of gonorrhea and not even know that he or she has a sexually transmitted disease. (See chapter 10 about treatment.) A single painful, swollen knee will lead to diagnosis of the underlying sexually transmitted disease.

LYME DISEASE

When undetected and untreated, Lyme disease can lead to inflammation that causes arthritis-like pain and swelling in the knees. This can happen to both children and adults. This condition is explained in detail in chapter 11.

BLOUNT'S DISEASE

Bobby was the youngest of three boys each born a year apart. A happy and inquisitive baby, Bobby began walking before he was a year old. His parents thought he simply wanted to keep up with his two brothers. But as the boys got older, the parents noticed that Bobby's legs bowed at an awkward angle and that sometimes he complained that his legs hurt.

All babies are born with bowed legs because of their position in the uterus. Some toddlers' legs can look as if they just got off a horse, but the legs straighten out as the child grows. It is normal for a child's knees to go from bowed to straight to knock-kneed (valgus) to the ultimate adult alignment. Bobby was diagnosed with a medical condition called Blount's disease, a growth disorder in which the inner part of the tibia, just below the knee, grows at a slower rate than the outer part. In children under age two, it is not easy to distinguish between normal bowed legs and Blount's disease, but if the disease is discovered early, it can be treated with bracing.

Blount's disease occurs both in young children and adolescents. Medical scientists suspect that it is caused by the effect of weight on the growth plate and may be associated with obesity and early walking. In contrast to physiologic (normal) bowing, Blount's disease gets progressively worse and can cause severe bowing in one or both legs if not treated. It is more common among African-American children, but there is not a known genetic factor that causes this disease. (See chapter 11 about diagnosis and treatment.)

BONE CANCER

Most cancer in the bones is secondary cancer (metastasis) in adults that has spread from other parts of the body. Cancer that begins in the bone is rare—comprising fewer than 0.2 percent of all cancers—but it is more common in children than in adults. According to the American Cancer Society, about 2,750 new cases of primary bone cancer were diagnosed in 2005.

Primary bone cancer can occur in any one of your body's 206 bones but most commonly occurs in the long bones of your arms and legs. In certain cases, primary bone cancer can be traced to exposure to radiation. While routine X-rays won't harm you, extended doses of radiation (from treatment for other cancers, for example) may add to the risk of developing bone cancer. This is especially true if the radiotherapy was given while a child's bones were still growing. However, as radiation treatment has become more sophisticated and precise, such side effects have been greatly reduced.

Pain is the most common alert to bone cancer, along with swelling and tenderness. Cancer can weaken the bones, making them more vulnerable to fracture. Often an injury will bring a child to the doctor, where an X-ray will reveal an abnormality of bone. Other possible signs of bone cancer include fever, weight loss, night pain, fatigue, and anemia.

The types of primary bone cancer that can affect the knee include:

Osteogenic sarcoma, also called osteosarcoma, grows in the bone tissue and is the most common type of primary bone cancer. It affects adolescents and young adults and usually occurs in the long bones such as the femur and tibia. Osteosarcoma is more common in males than females. It has been suggested that repeated trauma to an area may be a risk factor for developing this type of cancer, but it remains unclear. Cancer in bone can make the area weaker and more susceptible to trauma. A subsequent injury will bring a child to the attention of a physician, at which point the diagnosis is then made. Genetics may also play a role in the development of osteosarcoma. Children and adults with other inherited abnormalities such as multiple bony growths (exostoses), are at increased risk for osteosarcoma.

Ewing's sarcoma grows from the bone marrow tissue, found mainly in the hollow middle part of bones of the hips, ribs, and thighs. (Other cancers that arise in the bone marrow, such as leukemia, multiple myeloma, and lymphoma, are not considered bone cancers, but they do affect the bone and may require orthopedic management.) Ewing's sarcoma is the second most common malignant tumor in children and young adults and occurs most often between ages ten and twenty. The number of males with Ewing's sarcoma is slightly higher than the number of females. (See chapter 11 about treatment of bone cancer.)

KEY POINTS

- Traumatic injury is a major cause of knee pain in adolescents, especially those involved in organized sports.

- Osgood-Schlatter disease is an overuse injury that affects the growing bones of athletic young people whose long bones are growing rapidly.
- Osteochondritis dissecans (OCD) is related to the loss of blood supply to the knee cartilage. It is most common in adolescents and is also seen in young adults.
- Discoid meniscus can cause a clicking noise, knee pain, and locking in young children.
- Juvenile rheumatoid arthritis can cause knee pain in children.
- Blount's disease, a condition where the shin bows excessively, occurs both in young children and adolescents.
- Osteosarcoma and Ewing's sarcoma affect the long bones of the arms and legs and are more common in children than adults.

Chapter 5

Knee Pain in Adults

Throughout your adult life, you experience physical changes in eyesight, hearing, weight, bone density, and muscle strength. Your knees change too, and they may be more vulnerable to pain from particular types of injury or medical conditions at certain times. If you are aware, you may be able to prevent pain or modify the duration of your symptoms.

YOUNG ADULTS (AGES EIGHTEEN TO FORTY)

Young adults have busy lives, finishing college, starting careers and families, and making their mark on the world. They are not overly concerned about their later years, and you would be hard-pressed to find anyone in this group worried about what condition his or her knees will be in when they reach fifty. In adults between twenty and forty, knee pain is most commonly caused by trauma or from overuse injury, although less frequently it can be caused by a medical condition such as inflammatory arthritis or Lyme disease.

47

Traumatic knee injuries sustained by athletes and "weekend warriors" playing football, soccer, skiing, and basketball are common in this age group. They incur ligament sprains involving the ACL and MCL, as well as injury to both the meniscal and articular cartilage. Young adults who work hard over long hours during the week don't always warm up properly before their weekend sports workout. Ironically, those who exercise on a regular basis at their local health or fitness club can be prone to injury because they overdo their workouts or do them improperly. A sports injury, fall, or other accident may injure your knee tendons or cartilage, but the most common injuries seen in young adults are to the ligaments and the meniscus.

We have included adolescents in both the previous chapter and this one because there is overlap in the types of injuries seen, particularly in sports. Adolescent athletes are now competing with an intensity not seen in collegiate athletics twenty years ago. They may participate in multiple varsity sports or in a single sport with multiple games and training sessions.

Traumatic Ligament Injuries

You can sprain or tear one of your four knee ligaments if you twist your knee beyond the normal range of motion. This can occur when you pivot while your foot is planted in one place, when you slip or fall, or when you land badly after a jump. If you are an athlete, the injury might occur with a fall, colliding with another player on the field, or an off-balance twist. A ligament injury is likely to cause immediate mild-to-severe pain and discomfort that get worse when you walk or bend your knee.

The most frequently injured ligament is the anterior cruciate ligament (ACL), followed by the medical collateral ligament (MCL).

The **anterior cruciate ligament (ACL)** restrains the tibia from sliding forward on your femur, and, together with the other three knee ligaments, it works to provide stability as your knee rotates (see chapter 1). Whether you are casually turning as you walk or cutting side to side sharply in a basketball game, the ACL is critical to your knee's performance. This ligament gets a lot of attention because it is injured frequently and because an ACL injury in an athlete can result in a significant loss of playing time. Athletes injure the ACL when changing direction, jumping, or stopping suddenly. These injuries are most common in football, soccer, basketball, lacrosse, skiing, field hockey, and volleyball.

If you tear your ACL completely, you are likely to know it right away. You may feel or hear a pop in your knee and have intense pain and immediate swelling. You will feel your knee collapse and may have difficulty standing on the affected leg. Your knee may buckle if you try to walk. In rare cases or when there is only a partial ACL injury, you may not feel significant pain immediately, and your knee won't feel as unstable. However, within two to twelve hours, your knee will swell considerably and hurt when you try to stand or bend it. If you try to continue cutting-and-pivoting activities on an injured ACL, you run the risk of damaging the cartilage in your knee. Without proper treatment, ACL injury can result in chronic knee instability.

Posterior cruciate ligament (PCL) sprains and tears are not as common as ACL injuries. The PCL, which crosses from the front of the femur to the back of the tibia, behind your knee, is most commonly injured by a fall on a bent knee or a blow to the front of the knee during a contact sport or in a car accident when your knee strikes the dashboard. The impact drives the tibia backward relative to the femur. This can result in pain and swelling, and your knee may feel unstable. If the laxity is severe, it can eventually lead to arthritis in the medial and patellofemoral compartments of the knee. The thin, smooth articular cartilage in the medial and patellofemoral compartments can wear, which, in turn, results in localized arthritis of the knee.

The **medial collateral ligament (MCL)** connects your femur to your tibia and provides stability to the inner side of your knee. Injuries to this ligament are usually caused by a blow to the outside of the knee, or if you slip and fall with your foot sliding out to the side. This is a frequent injury in football and skiing. MCL injury is usually accompanied by sharp pain and sometimes a ripping sensation along the inside of your knee. You may hear a pop at the time of injury, and your knee will swell over the next twelve to twenty-four hours.

The **lateral collateral ligament (LCL),** which connects your femur to the fibula and stabilizes the outer side, is the least frequently injured knee ligament. Injury is likely to result from a collision when the knee is forced out away from the body or is struck on the inside corner, driving the joint into a bowlegged position. This ligament can also be injured with knee hyperextension. An example of this would be sliding into a base during a baseball game with your knee locked straight.

Meniscus Injuries

The menisci, those two C-shaped cartilage pads that sit between the femur and the tibia in each knee joint, can be injured when you twist quickly or rotate your upper leg while your foot remains fixed, such as when you pivot to hit a tennis ball.

The seriousness of a tear depends on its location, extent, and your age. In adolescents and young adults, meniscus tears are generally caused by significant trauma. Tears in people over age forty often have a degenerative component. In this case, the meniscus has been weakened by age and tears with much less trauma.

You may not initially notice a small meniscus tear, but pain and mild to moderate swelling may develop within twenty-four to forty-eight hours. A small tear could occur in a young person with a twisting or hyper-flexion injury such as a fall or during contact in sports. In an older person, a tear could occur with a misstep or something as simple as squatting deeply to pick something up.

Meniscus tears come in a variety of shapes and sizes, which are reflected in the symptoms that they cause. For example, the cartilage may tear lengthwise or from the inside to the outside rim of the meniscus. This is known as a radial tear. Sometimes a large lengthwise tear can move into the center of the knee joint instead of staying around the joint's edge. This is called a bucket-handle tear. A flap of the torn meniscus can interfere with knee movement and cause your knee joint to lock so that you can't straighten it completely.

Generally, when you injure your meniscus, you feel some pain, particularly when you try to bend or straighten your knee. If the pain is mild, it's safe to continue moving, but when there is severe pain or limitation of motion, there's a chance that a fragment of the meniscus is caught between the femur and the tibia.

Pain and swelling are common with acute injuries and will often resolve within weeks, but they are likely to return when you are active again. In addition, repeated injuries can increase the size and severity of existing tears. This is particularly true for flap tears, which can get caught in the knee and increase in size.

After any meniscus injury, your knee may swell, click, lock, feel weak, or give way. Symptoms may disappear on their own, but they frequently return and require treatment. Sometimes a previous meniscus injury can become painful months or even years later, particularly if your knee is injured a second time.

Iliotibial Band (ITB) Syndrome

Overuse injuries are common in this age group. You remember Cheryl from chapter 2, who was so overly zealous with her training for the city marathon that she developed iliotibial band syndrome. Cheryl's mistake was doing too much, too soon. Rather than pace her training, she increased it rapidly, raising both her speed and her mileage at the same time. She continued to train despite pain and neglected her stretching. The result was terrible pain on the outside of her knees.

This common cause of lateral knee pain in runners and cyclists is the result of a combination of overuse and tightness of the iliotibial band, a long, strong structure that runs along the outside of the thigh to the shin. This syndrome is common in distance runners and cyclists and can cause a sharp, burning pain or a dull ache along the outer side of the knee. Pain can begin ten to fifteen minutes into a run. Initially, the pain goes away with rest, but if not treated properly it can ultimately cause pain when you walk or go up and down stairs. (See chapter 9 about treatment.)

Patellofemoral Pain and Chondromalacia of the Patella

Patellofemoral pain occurs under and around the front of the kneecap. It is poorly understood and can be the result of a variety of factors, including the misalignment of your kneecap, or inadequate muscle strength or flexibility. The misalignment can result from a kneecap that is too high (patella alta), too low (patella baja), tilted, or too loose.

Inflexible and tight muscles can increase the pressure at your patellofemoral joint, resulting in pain in the front of your knee. For example, overly tight hamstring muscles in the back of your thigh make it difficult to straighten your knee. As a result, the quadriceps in the front of your thigh have to create more force to extend the knee. This puts more stress on your kneecap. When your quadriceps are too tight, they can also increase pressure behind your kneecap. Tightness of the soft tissues on the outside of your leg, such as the iliotibial band and the supporting lateral retinaculum, can result in patellar tilt. This means that the patella tilts in the trochlear groove. This can increase the pressure on the undersurface of the lateral kneecap, bringing about inflammation and pain. Your quads help to hold your kneecap in a balanced position, so weakness of these muscles—particularly the one on the inside of your knee—can contribute to patellofemoral pain.

Weakness or tightness of the hip abductor muscles that

extend from your hip to your thigh and help you rotate your femur have also been implicated in patellofemoral pain. A physical therapist can teach you a variety of exercises that will progressively strengthen your hip and leg muscles while protecting your knee.

Patellofemoral pain may affect one or both knees, and it feels worse when you bend your knees while squatting, climbing stairs, or sitting for long periods of time. It is a common condition of active adults, especially runners (it is known as runner's knee) as well as skiers, cyclists, and soccer players. Young women who have a slight misalignment of the kneecap are also vulnerable. Patellofemoral pain may also be an early sign of arthritis in people who are overweight and out of condition.

The most frequent symptoms of patellofemoral pain are:

- A dull pain around or under the front of your knee that worsens when you get up from a prolonged period of sitting.
- Pain that worsens when you walk down hills or go down stairs.
- Mild swelling and tenderness of the knee.
- Pain when your knee is extended (straight), and you press your kneecap against the top of your femur.
- A grating or grinding sensation when you extend your knee.
- Gradual pain that increases over several weeks.

Chondromalacia of the patella has historically been used as an umbrella term for slowly progressive pain arising between the patella and the underlying trochlea, regardless of the cause. However, it actually describes a specific condition that begins as softening of the cartilage of the patella or trochlea and can progress to thinning of the cartilage and the development of patellofemoral arthritis (cartilage loss).

In young adults, chondromalacia, like patellofemoral pain, most often occurs because of poor alignment of the kneecap or as a result of injury, overuse, or muscle weakness. When the kneecap is not gliding smoothly across the trochlea, forces can concentrate on one area, resulting in overload and the ultimate breakdown or roughening of the underlying cartilage. Damage can range from a slightly abnormal cartilage surface to the complete loss of cartilage from the bone. When caused by an injury such as a fall or blow to the kneecap, a small piece of cartilage or a fragment containing a piece of bone (osteochondral fracture) can result in an irregular surface. Pain may come and go, but you feel it with squatting, kneeling, and negotiating steps, especially going down the stairs. In sports, you may feel pain with repeated bending of the knees.

Teenagers can get chondromalacia in response to excessive and uneven pressure because of structural changes in the legs with rapid growth and muscle imbalance around the knee. In young people, the loss of cartilage is uncommon, so the condition can be reversible. There may be mild softening or breakdown of cartilage. Thus, the term chondromalacia is not as accurate as anterior knee pain syndrome or patellofemoral stress syndrome. In most young people, pain comes and goes for a few years until they stop growing. People over forty, however, can develop chondromalacia as their cartilage thins with age or inflammation.

The most important thing about patellofemoral pain is determining the cause so that an appropriate treatment plan can be made. If you have significant pain on a daily basis, with or without swelling, you should be evaluated by a doctor. Because patellofemoral pain can be caused by patella soft tissue structures that are too tight or too loose, or by muscles that are too taut or excessively lax, it is important to be evaluated for all of the potential causes of anterior knee pain in order to find an effective strategy for treatment. The knee pain and inflammation can actually cause your quadriceps to weaken further. Then you get caught in a cycle of lost strength and pain that limits your activity.

Quadriceps and Patellar Tendinitis

Runners, skiers, cyclists, and jumping athletes are vulnerable to quadriceps and patellar tendinitis. This can occur from inflammation or degeneration of the tendons that connect the quadriceps muscles to the patella and the patella to the tibia. It is believed to be caused by repeated stress to those tendons. For example, if you ride a bike every day for many miles, you may overload these tendons. This can be exacerbated by a poor-fitting bike. If the seat and pedals are not adjusted to suit your height properly, excessive pressure can be placed on the patella, and the quadriceps and patella tendons.

The quadriceps tendon attaches to the top of the kneecap and then merges with the connective tissue overlying the kneecap. This tissue continues down to join with the patellar tendon, which attaches to the tibia, so it functions like one long tendon with two sections that help your muscles move your knee. When these tendons are injured or subject to overuse, microtears develop and can result in inflammation. Sometimes rest and ice applications can relieve this pain in its early stages. Over time the condition progresses to tendinosis, with degeneration and scar formation in the tendons. Tendinosis is degeneration of the tendons with damage to tissues at a cellular level. In more serious cases, surgery may be needed to repair the tendons.

Injury to the patella tendon can also occur with blunt trauma, such as a fall on a bent knee or a dashboard injury. This may result in a partial tear to the patella tendon that may cause symptoms with daily activity. (See chapter 8 about treatment.)

Pigmented Villonodular Synovitis (PVNS)

Jean is a twenty-four-year-old graduate history student who is in good shape and exercises regularly. She spends a good deal of time in her university library, and while walking through the book stacks, her knee would occasionally feel stiff. One day, a clicking noise developed. Jean did not remember injuring her knee and thought perhaps it was from so much sitting and reading. To combat this, she increased her evening bike rides and running. However, her knee began to swell, and she noticed a mobile lump just above her kneecap. At last, her knee locked in a bent position, and Jean had to be helped out of the library.

Jean's doctor found that she had pigmented villonodular synovitis, a benign tumor that arises from the synovial tissue that lines the knee and causes pain and swelling. It is uncommon, occurring only in two in every one million persons, and affects primarily young adults between twenty and forty. While it is considered locally aggressive, PVNS rarely spreads to the bones outside the affected joint. The knee is the most common site for PVNS, and although the tumors are benign, they can cause significant knee disability.

For unknown reasons, the synovium undergoes change when affected by PVNS and becomes thick and overgrown. Your knee may swell, or you may feel a mobile mass and experience locking. A rust-colored iron pigment known as hemosiderin accumulates in the synovium along with large, foamy cells called giant cells. The overgrowth can occur diffusely throughout your knee by way of a generalized thickening of the entire lining (diffuse PVNS), or it can be localized and form a nodule that remains attached to the synovium by a stalk (nodular or pedunculated PVNS). Although PVNS does not metastasize, some cases are more locally aggressive and harder to treat.

Diffuse PVNS is more problematic because the thickened synovium is present throughout the knee joint. This type is difficult to remove surgically without affecting normal structures in the knee and has a much greater chance of recurring. However, if it is not treated, it can cause permanent damage to the knee joint and can lead to arthritis. With the isolated nodular form, you are more likely to have mechanical symptoms such as locking. This form is less likely to recur after surgery. (See chapter 11 about treatment.)

Rheumatoid Arthritis

Unlike osteoarthritis, which primarily affects the articular cartilage in your knee, rheumatoid arthritis begins in the synovial tissue. Rheumatoid arthritis (RA) is an autoimmune disorder, which means the body mistakenly identifies some of its own cells and tissues as foreign. The immune system, which normally helps to fight off harmful foreign substances such as bacteria or viruses, begins to attack healthy cells and tissues. The result is inflammation characterized by redness, heat, pain, and swelling.

RA is two to three times more common in women and most frequently begins between the ages of twenty and fifty. However, it sometimes strikes older adults and can also affect children in the form of juvenile rheumatoid arthritis (see chapter 4). You may also be at risk for RA if you were exposed to a bacterium or virus that acted as a trigger if you already have an inherited susceptibility.

RA is the most debilitating form of arthritis and can affect almost any joint in your body, including your knees. It usually affects both knees at the same time. Sonja, a young schoolteacher, developed RA in both knees by the time she was thirty-five but was able to reduce pain with medication and exercise. Although it is a chronic disease, RA tends to vary in severity and can go through flare-ups that alternate with periods of remission. In addition to pain and swelling, you are likely to have aching and stiffness, especially when you get up in the morning or after periods of inactivity; loss of motion in your knees and the potential for deformity of your knee joints may also occur over time. A low-grade fever and a general malaise sometimes occur with RA, as this is a systemic disease. There is no cure for RA, but it can be treated to minimize pain and disease progression. (See chapter 10 about treatment.)

Psoriatic Arthritis

You won't get psoriatic arthritis unless you have psoriasis, but just because you have psoriasis doesn't mean that you will get this type of arthritis. Psoriatic arthritis affects the joints of adults (and sometimes children) with psoriasis, a skin condition that causes patches of thick, red skin to form on certain areas of the body. Both psoriasis and arthritis are autoimmune conditions, caused when the body's immune system begins to attack healthy cells and tissue. The majority of people have symptomatic skin lesions before they are diagnosed with arthritis. It is most common between the ages of thirty and fifty, generally affecting men and women equally, although some rare forms are gender specific. The severe form of psoriatic arthritis is more common at a younger age and in women and those with sudden-onset joint pain.

Psoriatic arthritis may affect one joint or many with pain, swelling, and a feeling of warmth to the touch. Pain can range from mild to severe, but signs and symptoms change as the disease continues. It can be debilitating and painful, and despite treatment, it can eventually erode the joint. It is difficult to estimate how many people have this form of arthritis, but according to Mayo Clinic statistics, approximately 10 percent to 15 percent of people with psoriasis will eventually develop psoriatic arthritis.

In addition, if you have a close relative with the disease, you may be more vulnerable. Medical scientists suspect that the cause is both genetic and environmental. Certain gene mutations appear to be associated with psoriatic arthritis. But having the mutation alone may not cause you to have this condition. Like rheumatoid arthritis, there may also be some physical or environmental trigger such as a viral or bacterial infection that results in disease if you have the inherited tendency.

Doctors have identified patterns in which psoriatic arthritis occurs, and most people move from one pattern to another during their lifetime.

Asymmetric psoriatic arthritis usually affects joints on only one side of your body or different joints on each side. This is the mildest form of the disease. One to three joints are involved, such as the knee, hip, or elbow.

Symmetric psoriatic arthritis usually affects four or more of the same joints on both sides of your body. More women than men have this type, and the psoriasis associated with this condition tends to be severe. The arthritis is similar to but milder than rheumatoid arthritis, which is also more common in women. And like rheumatoid arthritis, it can cause permanent damage to the joint. (See chapter 10 about treatment.)

MIDDLE AGE (AGES FORTY TO SIXTY)

Time is catching up. In addition to the problems experienced during your twenties to forties, new causes of knee pain can arise as you grow older. Any knee injury sustained earlier in life has the potential to intensify now. In your forties, you begin to lose muscle mass at a rate of about 1 percent a year. With less muscle, the knee joint, tendons, and ligaments have to absorb more of the force of walking and other daily activities. Your knees' articular cartilage may begin to thin out over the years and become less resilient. Any extra weight you are carrying puts more strain on your knees. According to one survey, more than a quarter of women over forty report having knee pain most days, and even more report persistent pain after fifty. If you have not paid attention, now is the time to get serious about getting into shape and protecting your knees from pain and disability. (See chapter 18 about conditioning.)

Tendon Injuries

Tendon injuries are most common between the ages of forty and seventy and are uncommon in younger adults. However, patellar tendon tears can occur in young athletes with significant knee trauma and can occur in combination with complete MCL and ACL tears.

Tendons are the thick, fibrous cords that attach muscles to bone. Injuries to tendons can range from repetitive overuse injury such as tendinitis (inflammation of a tendon) to a ruptured or completely torn tendon. When you overuse a tendon while dancing, cycling, running, or skiing, it becomes inflamed or sustains small partial tears. This results in tendinitis or tendinosis of the patellar tendon that connects the patella to the tibia or the quadriceps tendon that attaches the quadriceps muscle to the patella. Tendinitis and tendinosis are both overuse injuries.

If your quadriceps tendon or patellar tendon ruptures, either partially or completely, the pain is likely to be intense at the time of injury or if you try to extend your knee. If the tendon is completely ruptured, you won't be able to extend your knee fully. The most common mechanism for a tear of either the quadriceps or patellar tendon is falling with your knee bent, because two forces are acting in opposite directions. When you bend your knee, the muscle tendon unit is lengthening to accommodate the bend. But it is also "firing," or shortening, to try to stabilize the knee. (See chapter 8 about treatment.)

Gout

When Len's doctor told him that gout was causing the knee pain that frequently bothered him in the middle of the night, he was shocked. He thought gout was a Victorian disease. At forty-five, Len did not consider himself old, but he was definitely developing a middle-aged spread. A winemaker by profession, Len tasted wine— mostly red wines—daily, but didn't drink them, at least not then. However, he also sponsored lavish dinners for potential distributors and other guests of the vineyard, so he drank a good deal of the wine, and these dinners often included foods such as foie gras, fish and game, sweetbreads, and mushrooms from the local forest. Len soon learned that all of these foods contain purines, which play a role in the development of gout. Purines are natural substances found in your body as well as in foods, but in some types of foods, such as organ meats, they are present in higher concentrations.

Men from forty to fifty are more vulnerable than women to get gout, one of the most acutely painful rheumatic diseases. Gout is caused by deposits of needlelike crystals of uric acid in connective tissues of the knee. It is also called crystal-induced arthritis and causes sudden severe pain and swelling. It is a type of inflammatory arthritis, which can result in joint stiffness. Gout can cause intense pain in the lower extremities, with the big toe and knee affected 75 percent of the time. Gout can also affect the midfoot, ankles, heels, knees, wrists, fingers, and elbows. Pain comes on suddenly—often at night—and without warning. Swelling and redness also develop. The discomfort subsides over one to two weeks, leaving your knee joint apparently normal and pain free.

Up to 18 percent of those with gout have a family history of the disease, but there are other risk factors for developing gout. These include being overweight, drinking too much alcohol, and eating too many foods rich in purines. Gout re-

---

GOT GOUT? AVOID THESE

Foods High in Purines

Organ meats such as liver and kidneys
Fish such as anchovies, sardines, herring, cod, trout, haddock, mussels, and scallops
Bacon
Veal
Game such as venison and turkey
Alcohol (especially beer and red wine)

Foods Moderately High in Purines

Asparagus, spinach, and mushrooms
Kidney beans, lentils, lima beans
Beef, ham, pork
Chicken and duck
Shellfish such as crab, lobster, oysters, shrimp
Bouillon made from anything on this list

---

sults from an excess of uric acid that is deposited in specific joints. Uric acid is a waste product that results from the breakdown of purines, which are part of all human tissue and are found in many foods, such as liver (foie gras), organ meats (sweetbreads), fish and game, mushrooms, and legumes (see page 64 for a list). Some medications, such as diuretics or anti-inflammatory medicines such as aspirin, may also be causative factors.

Normally, uric acid is dissolved in the blood, passed through the kidneys, and eliminated in the urine. If the body increases its production of uric acid, or if the kidneys do not eliminate enough from the body, it builds up in the blood. This is called hyperuricemia. Hyperuricemia is not a disease and by itself is not dangerous. However, if as a result of hyperuricemia, excess uric acid crystals form, the excess builds up in the joint spaces, causing inflammation. Uric acid deposits can appear as lumps under the skin around the joints and at the rim of the ear. These crystals can also collect in the kidneys and cause kidney stones. While the body processes uric acid continuously, it is not clear why the pain and swelling associated with gout occurs so frequently at night.

Gout can progress through four stages:

1. Asymptomatic: No symptoms, but with high levels of uric acid in the blood—hyperuricemia.
2. Acute gout or acute gouty arthritis: Uric acid crystals deposit in joint spaces, causing a sudden onset of intense pain and swelling in the joints. An acute attack commonly occurs at night and can be triggered by stress, alcohol (red wine in particular), drugs, or the presence of another illness. In early

stages of the disease, attacks usually subside within
three to ten days, even without treatment, and the
next attack may not occur for months or even
years. Over time, the attacks can last longer and
occur more frequently.

3. Interval or intercritical gout: This is the period
between acute attacks. In this stage, you don't
have any symptoms, and your knee joint functions normally.

4. Chronic tophaceous gout is the most disabling
stage of gout and usually develops over a long
period, such as ten years. In this stage, the disease
has caused permanent damage to the affected
joints and sometimes to the kidneys.

   With proper medical treatment, most cases
   of gout can be kept under control and won't
   progress to the advanced stage. (See chapter 10
   for treatment.)

Degenerative Meniscus Tears

Degenerative meniscus tears become increasingly common in people ages forty to sixty, as the meniscus becomes
less elastic and begins to break down. These tears can result
from something as ordinary as squatting or from a more
significant trauma. Such tears can cause insidious pain,
swelling, and stiffness. It is estimated that 50 percent of people over age fifty have abnormal menisci, many of which do
not cause symptoms.

Degenerative meniscus tears sometimes cause symptoms and other times are completely quiet. For example,
John, the bus driver in chapter 2, felt immediate pain when

he squatted down to assist a passenger in a wheelchair, but Josephine, fifty-five, discovered her torn meniscus by accident when she had surgery for another knee condition. The treatment of a degenerative meniscus tear is completely dependent on symptoms. Meniscus tears can be pain free or can cause local pain along the medial or lateral joint line. They can cause pain in the back of the knee when you climb stairs, squat—even bend your knee to put on your socks. Meniscus tears can also cause mechanical symptoms such as catching or locking. (See chapter 8 about treatment.)

MATURE ADULTS (AGES SIXTY AND OVER)

While osteoarthritis is the most common cause of knee pain in mature adults, in this age group you are also susceptible to pain caused by lack of flexibility and strength, as well as weakened bones.

Jane, Lillian, and Sue, friends since college, all planned to retire at the same time and travel the world together. Over the years, they met periodically to plan adventures like rafting the Colorado River, walking in a rain forest in Belize, even dogsledding in Alaska. Jane had begun to develop knee pain in her forties, but she simply avoided walking or doing anything that seemed to increase her pain. She was overweight and did not seek treatment for her knee pain, nor did she lose weight. In contrast, her friends kept active with bike riding and regular fitness workouts, including yoga. By the time all three women retired, Jane was diabetic, had high blood pressure, and was crippled with arthritis in her knees. Her medical conditions made getting a knee replacement more risky. Had Jane been more attentive to her health over the years, she might have been able to join her globetrotting friends instead of settling for postcards.

Osteoarthritis

Osteoarthritis is the major orthopedic reason that people become less mobile and more disabled with increasing age. Osteoarthritis is also called degenerative arthritis because the knee articular cartilage slowly wears away with increasing age. There may also be a genetic component, as certain families seem to develop osteoarthritis at an earlier age than the general population.

About 13 percent of the population—or thirty-five million people—are sixty-five and older, and more than half of them have evidence of osteoarthritis in at least one joint. The Centers for Disease Control and Prevention estimates that the number of arthritis cases will increase nearly 40 percent by 2030 when the number of people ages forty-five to sixty-five doubles due to the baby boomer generation growing older. The Arthritis Foundation reports that osteoarthritis is a serious and underestimated problem that affects about half the people sixty-five and over, primarily women. Aging, obesity, and injury contribute to what can be a crippling disease. The speed at which cartilage degenerates is likely dependent on a combination of factors, including age, gender, activity level, and obesity, and may in part be genetically determined. Individual cartilage biology, history of knee trauma, and knee alignment are part of the complex equation that determines who will and who won't develop osteoarthritis.

There are some anatomical factors that contribute to osteoarthritis. Being loose jointed (ligament laxity), knock-kneed, or bowlegged can result in uneven forces on the cartilage and meniscus. Being loose jointed means that the ligaments that support your knee are too lax. This may increase your risk of patellar instability and development of patellofemoral arthritis. Being knock-kneed (valgus alignment) means that your knees bend inward and point toward each other when you are standing straight up. This alignment results in increased force on the outside compartment of the knee. Being bowlegged (varus alignment) means your legs curve outward when you stand (think of the cowboys in the movies!). This alignment places increased load on the inside, or medial compartment, of the knee.

A difference in the length of your legs can affect your susceptibility to osteoarthritis. According to a 2006 study at the Thurston Arthritis Research Center at the University of North Carolina at Chapel Hill, even a slight difference in leg length may add to your risk. The study, presented at a conference of the American College of Rheumatology, involved more than three thousand volunteers, including 210 who had a difference in leg lengths of two centimeters (about one inch) or more. This small difference is seldom noticed because people compensate for it in the way they walk. The study suggests that using orthotic devices such as shoe lifts to equalize leg length may prevent the disease or keep it from getting worse.

Osteoarthritis develops gradually, causing varying degrees of pain and swelling. At first you might have some localized soreness when you run, jump, or participate in other activities that put a high load on the knee. Over time, the pain may linger after the activity has ceased, and you may notice pain when walking and standing, even without engaging in high load activity.

Many people with osteoarthritis report increased symptoms with damp or cold weather. Scientists have yet to explain this patient perception and a possible link between pain and weather—and there are no scientific studies to support this perception—but some people describe pain that intensifies just before a storm, when atmospheric pressure drops.

If you have osteoarthritis, your knees may be more painful and stiff for the first half hour or so after you get up in the morning, or after you've been sitting for a long time. Pain can also occur when you are going up or down stairs. If you have cartilage loss, particularly at the patellofemoral joint, your knee may also feel unstable or feel like it is going to lock or catch.

Some professional athletes—football and soccer players, for example—develop osteoarthritis at an early age because of repetitive injury to their knee cartilage. There is special concern about young female athletes playing basketball and soccer today. With repeated injuries to the cartilage, meniscus, and ligaments, they may develop osteoarthritis similar to that seen in male athletes at an early age. A joint misalignment following trauma can lead to greater localized load on the cartilage, which can accelerate the development of arthritis.

Today more adults run, play sports, and maintain a highly active lifestyle than did previous generations. There is no scientific data that an active lifestyle in the absence of knee injury will speed up degeneration of knee cartilage. If you have had a cartilage or meniscus injury, low-impact sports may be a more sensible way to stay physically active.

But keep in mind that osteoarthritis is a disease, not necessarily a condition of old age. (See chapter 10 about treatment.)

Pseudogout

Pseudogout is sometimes confused with gout because it produces similar symptoms of pain, swelling, and inflammation that can last for days or weeks. However, pseudogout is caused by an excess of calcium pyrophosphate crystals, which deposit in the synovium. Pseudogout is also called chondrocalcinosis or calcium pyrophosphate deposition disease (CPPD). Pseudogout affects larger joints of arms and legs, typically the knees of older adults, although, unlike gout, it does not affect the big toe. It can be present in some people with osteoarthritis, though these is no clear link that proves it causes arthritis. While the calcium pyrophosphate crystals often deposit in areas of degenerative cartilage or a meniscus, it is unclear if these crystals actually cause degeneration.

Age is the most common risk factor for pseudogout, followed by a history of prior knee injuries. Because the condition sometimes runs in families, genetic factors may play a role. If excess calcium is stored in your blood, it may be due to an underactive thyroid or an overactive parathyroid gland. Low magnesium levels in the diet may also be a factor. Magnesium is found in legumes, peanut butter, spinach, and some other dark green vegetables. (See chapter 10 about treatment.)

Bone Cancer

When cancer affects the bones of adults, it is usually a secondary cancer that has spread from another part of the body such as the lungs or breast. Primary bone cancer, typically affecting the long bones of arms or legs, strikes a small number of people each year, most of them children (see chapter 4). However, chondrosarcoma, a tumor of the cartilage that usually occurs around the knee, pelvis, or hip, is most common in adults over fifty and accounts for 26 percent of cases.

Some rarer types of bone cancer include fibrosarcoma, which appears in the knee or hip and can arise in older people after radiation therapy for other cancers. Giant-cell tumors usually begin in the knee and affect younger adults—women more than men.

It is suspected that adults with Paget's disease (a condition that causes normal bone cells to be replaced with abnormal bone cells) may be at increased risk for osteosarcoma. In some rare cases, a familial connection may put you at risk. For example, people with Li-Fraumeni syndrome, a rare predisposition to cancer at a young age, are at risk for many cancers, including osteosarcoma. People with Rothmund-Thomson syndrome, which causes short stature and skeletal problems, are also at risk for developing bone cancer. Hereditary retinoblastoma is a rare cancer of the eye, and children with this disease are also at increased risk for osteosarcoma. Another condition, multiple hereditary exostoses (abnormal growths on the bone surface), also increases the risk of developing a chondrosarcoma.

KEY POINTS

- Traumatic knee injuries are common among active young adults.
- Overuse injuries such as iliotibial band (ITB) syndrome and runner's knee are common among young adults.
- Pigmented villonodular synovitis (PVNS), a benign tumor of the synovial tissue, causes knee pain and swelling primarily in young adults.
- Rheumatoid arthritis frequently begins between ages twenty and fifty.
- Tendon injuries are most common in middle age.
- Gout causes knee pain mostly in middle-aged men.
- Degenerative meniscal tears become increasingly common in people between forty and sixty.
- Osteoarthritis, the loss and degeneration of articular cartilage, is the major orthopedic reason people become less mobile and more disabled as they get older.
- Pseudogout is more common in people over sixty-five, and may or may not cause pain.
- Primary bone cancer is rare, but people with certain medical conditions can be genetically predisposed to develop it.

Chapter 6

Finding the Doctor Who's Right for You

Eleanor had always been very careful about her health. She went to the doctors in her health maintenance organization (HMO) for regular checkups. When she was fifty-nine, Eleanor felt pain in her left knee, especially when bending or straightening it. Her primary care physician told her that she was simply getting older, and this was to be expected. He suggested she take a nonsteroidal anti-inflammatory drug (NSAID) and keep off her feet as much as she could. Eleanor did what he told her, but her knee did not get better. She lived in a rural community with few doctors. In addition, Eleanor was timid about questioning the doctor, even though she knew that he was not trained in orthopedics. Had Eleanor asked some questions, gone for a second opinion, or just insisted that her doctor dig deeper to find the cause of her pain, she might not have suffered for so long. Her friends convinced her to seek a specialist in a neighboring city. Eleanor learned that her pain had been caused by cartilage fragments that had come loose and interfered with her knee function. In a simple arthroscopic operation, the surface of the cartilage was smoothed, and cartilage fragments were removed. Eleanor was able to live without knee pain for many years to come.

Medicine is an ever-changing science, and this certainly applies to orthopedic care. New technologies are developed every year to help diagnose and treat knee injuries. New medications appear at regular intervals. Hospital stays are shortening, and, increasingly, testing and care are being rendered in the outpatient setting. The application of arthroscopy for the surgical treatment of joint injury and disease has opened new horizons in treatment. The surgical management of degenerative joint disease such as arthritis has changed tremendously over the last twenty to thirty years, as have doctors' abilities to replace a diseased joint with a prosthetic device (total joint replacement).

If you are in pain, you want to have access to the best and latest care that modern medicine has to offer. This will mean seeking care from a well-trained, board-certified physician or surgeon who participates in continuing medical education on a regular basis. Continuing education keeps doctors' knowledge fresh and up-to-date. These physicians may be on the staff of a university teaching hospital, a large urban or suburban medical center, or in practice in a small community. Such doctors will likely be affiliated with other physicians and physical therapists who are similarly trained and credentialed.

PHYSICIANS WHO TREAT KNEE PAIN

Most primary care physicians are internists or family practitioners who can treat knee pain resulting from a minor injury. However, you may need to see a specialist, such as an orthopedic surgeon or rheumatologist, if your pain and discomfort persist. Your primary care physician should refer you if the diagnosis is unclear or beyond his or her area of expertise, as Eleanor's doctor should have done. Knee pain may also be diagnosed and treated by physiatrists (physical medicine and rehabilitation specialists) or primary care physicians with additional training in musculoskeletal medicine. For example, a rheumatologist may manage the medical treatment of osteoarthritis or inflammatory arthritis before referring you to an orthopedic surgeon for arthroscopy or joint replacement. A primary care sports-medicine physician may manage an acute knee ligament injury prior to referral to an orthopedic surgeon for ligament reconstruction. An orthopedist may diagnose a stress fracture and then refer you to a primary care physician for treatment of underlying osteoporosis.

Orthopedic Surgeons

Orthopedic surgery is a surgical specialty for the diagnosis, care, and treatment of people with injuries and diseases of the musculoskeletal system. The doctors trained in this discipline are called orthopedists or orthopedic surgeons, as all orthopedists are orthopedic surgeons. Orthopedic surgery training consists of five years of postgraduate residency training and is commonly followed by specialty fellowship training in a particular discipline such as sports medicine, joint replacement, or hand, foot, or spine surgery. Orthopedists treat common injuries such as fractures, torn ligaments, dislocations, sprains, tendon injuries, meniscus and cartilage injuries, and stress fractures, as well as arthritis and medical or developmental conditions that cause knee pain. They employ medical, physical, and rehabilitative methods as well as surgery to restore function.

Some orthopedists confine their practices to specific areas of the musculoskeletal system, focusing solely on the spine, hip, foot, hand, shoulder, or knee. Still others practice specific subspecialties such as sports medicine, pediatric orthopedics, or joint replacement surgery.

Sports Medicine Specialists

Because so many knee injuries are the result of competitive sports, many orthopedists, primary care physicians, and physiatrists specialize in sports medicine and may work as a group sharing the care of patients. A sports medicine center can provide specialty sports-medicine care for active people of all ages and include staff with expertise not only in orthopedics, primary care sports medicine, and physiatry, but also psychology, nutrition, and exercise physiology.

Rheumatologists

Rheumatologists evaluate and treat arthritis and osteoporosis, and disorders in the bones, joints, or muscles related to these conditions. This includes diseases in which the body's immune system has turned against itself, with crippling, painful consequences such as rheumatoid arthritis, lupus, Sjogren's syndrome, and psoriatic arthritis. They also treat conditions such as Lyme disease, fibromyalgia, and muscle, joint, and bone pain. Rheumatologists utilize medications and physical therapy to cure acute musculoskeletal conditions of the knee or to help people manage chronic musculoskeletal conditions.

Physiatrists

Physiatrists specialize in rehabilitation of the musculoskeletal and nervous systems and have skills in electrodiagnostic testing, exercise methods, artificial or prosthetic limbs, bracing, and the use of selective injections. They can diagnose and oversee physical therapy and work with orthopedists in the management of a variety of conditions. The role of physiatry in the care of musculoskeletal conditions has expanded rapidly in the last decade.

Orthopedic Oncologists

An oncologist specializes in the treatment of cancer. Teams of medical and surgical orthopedic oncologists provide care to patients with primary or secondary tumors of the musculoskeletal system, including radiation and chemotherapy as needed. As mentioned in chapter 4, primary bone cancer (and metastasized cancer) may occur in the long bones of young people, often presenting as bone pain near the knee.

FINDING AN ORTHOPEDIST

Your primary care physician may be able to recommend one or more orthopedic surgeons, but it is a good idea to do some additional research on your own to find a doctor with whom you feel comfortable. A trusting relationship between doctor and patient is essential. Ask other doctors for their recommendations. Who do they see or who would they send a family member to see? Speak with people who have experience with orthopedic problems about how effective their treatment was, what they liked or disliked about the treatment or the doctor. Many people go from one doctor to another until they find someone who can help them. Some are reluctant to "doctor shop" effectively. Often, people insured with HMOs look in their health care directory and hope for the best.

Consult more knowledgeable sources such as professional medical associations, like your state medical society, books like this one, the internet, and other people who have had treatment. Ask them which hospitals and doctors have the best reputations for treating your condition, and which ones will accept your medical insurance. A team of physicians in the same hospital don't necessarily work with the same insurance plans. You may find one who will work with your plan, and this way you'll have access to the medical center you prefer.

You may also challenge the health-care system and become well informed. If you call your health insurance provider and ask where you can find a doctor who specializes in orthopedics, your provider will likely ask you for your zip code, assuming that you won't want to go far from home to find a doctor. Today many people travel to a distant city for treatment because they feel that a particular hospital or medical center will provide them with better, more advanced care than their local facility. Some medical centers even have hotel facilities for temporary housing.

Your state medical society and the American Medical Association (AMA) have physician referral services to help you locate a specialist. Also check with the Arthritis Foundation, American Academy of Orthopaedic Surgeons, and American Orthopaedic Society for Sports Medicine. (The appendix in the back of this book has a list of these sources.) Another well-respected but lesser-known physician listing site is the Castle Connolly Medical website, which has a "Find a Doctor" link (see appendix). This is a bit like the Zagat ratings of restaurants. Physician profiles are selected after peer nomination, extensive research, and careful review and screening by its own physician-directed research team.

Most states have a department of education that will provide records of a doctor's licensing. To find out if a specialist is accredited, check with the American Board of Medical Specialties. If you have any concerns, you can check with your state department of health to find out if the doctor has been the subject of any disciplinary action.

Choose a doctor who not only demonstrates compassion and the ability to listen but possesses up-to-date knowledge and experience dealing with your specific problem. Be sure to ask about the doctor's hospital affiliations, hours, availability, and health insurance participation. If he or she does not participate in your insurance plan, what are the office policies for billing and payment? If you are uninsured, does the doctor or hospital have a program to provide care on a sliding payment scale?

TOP TWENTY ORTHOPEDIC MEDICAL CENTERS IN THE UNITED STATES IN 2007

1. Hospital for Special Surgery (New York City, New York)
2. Mayo Clinic (Rochester, Minnesota)
3. Massachusetts General Hospital (Boston, Massachusetts)
4. Cleveland Clinic (Cleveland, Ohio)
5. Johns Hopkins Hospital (Baltimore, Maryland)
6. Duke University Medical Center (Durham, North Carolina)
7. New York-Presbyterian University Hospital of Columbia and Cornell (New York City, New York)
8. Rush University Medical Center (Chicago, Illinois)
9. UCLA Medical Center (Los Angeles, California)
10. New York University Hospital for Joint Diseases (New York City, New York)
11. Brigham and Women's Hospital (Boston, Massachusetts)
12. University of Pittsburgh Medical Center (Pittsburgh, Pennsylvania)
13. Thomas Jefferson University Hospital (Philadelphia, Pennsylvania)
14. Barnes-Jewish Hospital/Washington University (St. Louis, Missouri)
15. University of Washington Medical Center (Seattle, Washington)
16. University of Iowa Hospitals and Clinics (Iowa City, Iowa)
17. New England Baptist Hospital (Boston, Massachusetts)
18. Northwestern Memorial Hospital (Chicago, Illinois)
19. University Hospitals Case Medical Center (Cleveland, Ohio)
20. University of Michigan Hospitals and Health System (Ann Arbor, Michigan)

U.S. News & World Report ranking, 2007.

PAYING FOR THE BEST TREATMENT

If you have chronic knee pain that is difficult to diagnose and treat, you may want to visit several doctors before making a final decision about treatment. Most health insurance plans will pay for second opinions, which are always advised if your condition requires surgery. It's crucial to understand what is covered by your insurance plan before you see your doctor, because you may need diagnostic tests, surgical procedures or medications, and physical therapy. Not all of these options are covered equally by all plans.

Diagnostic testing, such as a high quality MRI (magnetic resonance imaging) scan, may not be available through your plan, especially if your plan is an HMO with a limited roster of doctors and medical facilities. Plans that allow you to choose your own doctors and facilities may cost you a considerable amount of additional money. However, there are ways of finding better care even within an HMO. For example, if you live in an area with a highly respected hospital or medical center known for its quality orthopedic department, find out if any of its doctors are included in your plan. At large centers, you may find some who are.

Use your insurer's website to find doctors who are authorized and may work in other parts of your city or even in other cities. You can also request doctors who work under the umbrella of a particular hospital that you feel comfortable with. Find out about the hospital's orthopedic specialists and their diagnostic testing services. Are they covered by your plan? If not, and if you do not need emergency treatment, you may be able to switch plans to one that will cover your needed tests and treatment.

INTERVIEWING POTENTIAL DOCTORS

If you have a serious knee injury, chronic knee pain, or you are contemplating surgery, you should arrange a face-to-face consultation. Bring any diagnostic tests, medical summaries, or prior operative reports with you. The physician will want to review any X-rays or test results that you have to help her determine if she can help you. If you are uncertain about the expertise of your physician, you might want to ask these kinds of questions:

- *How many patients with my physical complaint have you treated?* You want a doctor with considerable experience who is comfortable and competent treating your condition.
- *What are the short-term and long-term risks of treatment with medications versus undergoing an invasive procedure?* Make sure your doctor gives you a full review of all possible risks, and balances them with the benefits of the treatment. For example, long-term use of pain medications can lead to other problems.
- *Were most patients with conditions like mine significantly relieved or cured of their knee pain?* It's important to have an honest discussion here because not everyone is cured, and some patients may not follow their doctor's instructions for rehabilitation and lifestyle changes.
- *How do the long-term results of this treatment compare with results published by other doctors using the same methods in similar patients?*

- *How long should I undergo conservative treatment before surgery?* (There are more questions to ask about surgery in chapter 12.)
- *What lifestyle changes, including weight loss and alteration of exercise regimen and daily activities, should I try to relieve my knee pain before surgery?*

Be prepared for your visit. Ask in advance how much time is scheduled for you so that you can use the time well. If all of your questions can't be answered during the visit, ask the physician if she or her assistant will be able to speak with you or communicate via telephone, email, or mail at a later date.

If a doctor resists answering your questions, you may choose to change doctors. You should also understand that office visits are scheduled at standard intervals. If you know that you want or need more time, you should schedule it but also be willing to pay for the visit.

You should have your own plan B if your physician's proposed treatment plan proves ineffective or if you find that you have difficulty communicating with him or her about your treatment needs. If you seem to be getting nowhere with one doctor, you should consider finding another.

KEY POINTS

- Orthopedists are physicians who treat disorders of the musculoskeletal system. All orthopedists are orthopedic surgeons.

- Other physicians who treat knee pain include rheumatologists, physiatrists, pediatricians, and family practitioners.
- If you have any doubts about a doctor's ability to treat your knee pain effectively, or about the accuracy of the diagnosis, get a second opinion.
- Be as accurate as you can in describing your pain and the treatment(s) you have tried so far.
- Don't be afraid to check on a doctor's background and credentials.
- Investigate your health insurance coverage to find out how you can get the best quality medical treatment and diagnostic testing.

Chapter 7

Getting the Right Diagnosis

Medicine is a science, but there is an art to interpreting the signs and symptoms associated with your condition. It entails asking the right questions to uncover details in your lifestyle or medical history that might place you at risk for injury or that may produce symptoms. A physician should be sensitive to your story and be able to ask pertinent questions. The answers to these questions guide the physical examination, the diagnostic tests ordered, the diagnosis, and the initial treatment. In the limited resources of today's health care system, such time-consuming consultation is sometimes rare.

THE IMPORTANCE OF YOUR STORY

The history that you provide your doctor is a critical part of the diagnostic process. The more complete and detailed your information, the greater its value. Past and current illnesses are of great importance. Here are some examples: A history of cancer may be significant if you have new knee pain that cannot be blamed on a recent injury. Painful bursitis or tendinitis may have developed as a delayed complication from a fall or other injury suffered weeks or months before. Inflammatory arthritis of the knee and its resulting pain is sometimes associated with psoriasis (psoriatic arthritis). Medications that you take (for example, Lipitor, a drug for lowering cholesterol) can sometimes cause muscle pain.

Write things down before your visit and organize how you will describe your symptoms. List questions you want to ask. By thinking carefully about your knee pain, you will have organized information necessary to start the diagnostic process. Also, list your medicines and the names and addresses of your other health-care providers. If you have seen other physicians for evaluation of your condition, bring copies of their reports with you.

Here are some questions you should be prepared to answer:

How and When Did the Pain Begin?

Acute knee pain is often associated with a specific episode of trauma, such as pivoting your leg awkwardly during a sudden turn or hours spent kneeling in the garden. Acute pain from minor trauma often improves with time as the injured joint and surrounding muscles heal. Systemic illness, on the other hand, may cause pain that comes on gradually. People with inflammatory arthritis of the knee may have had some degree of stiffness and pain for six months or longer when first evaluated for their knee symptoms. Overuse injuries may be insidious in onset and are often related to increases in activity or changes in workout regimens, such as more or less exercise.

How Long Does the Pain Last, and Does It Recur?

This is relevant for pain that is episodic or fluctuates. When knee pain is caused by injury to your kneecap, the initial episode may resolve over a few days. However, with successive episodes, the pain may last longer and develop into a chronic pain disorder such as bursitis. With knee pain caused by a medical condition such as cancer or Lyme disease, rather than trauma, the important characteristics are both duration and frequency. This kind of knee pain is more persistent and, as in the case of a tumor, may last for months.

When Does Your Pain Occur, and What Makes It Feel Better or Worse?

Certain activities may provoke or reduce your knee pain. For example, you may have pain only when you stand or walk and feel fine when you sit down. Or you may have pain when you wake in the morning, but once you are moving around, it diminishes. Perhaps you have pain on the outside of your knee when you run, but it ends as soon as you stop. Going up or down stairs may provoke knee pain.

Have You Tried Over-the-Counter Medicines or Home Remedies?

If you have taken over-the-counter pain medications such as Advil, Tylenol, or Aleve, or nutritional supplements, you need to let your doctor know how much you take and for how long you have taken such medications. It is important to let the doctor know if these medications helped, for how long, whether you had any side effects from them, and whether you have tried other remedies such as applying ice or heat to the painful area.

Describe the Quality and Intensity of the Pain

Your doctor may ask you to grade the intensity of your knee pain on a scale of 0 to 10, with 0 being no pain and 10 being the worst possible pain. He or she will also want to know if the pain is sharp or dull, and whether a change of position causes it to increase or decrease.

Does Anyone in Your Family Have the Same Condition?

A strong family history of knee disorders may increase your risk of knee pain. Rheumatoid arthritis has a genetic predisposition, and so do some developmental anatomical conditions such as bowed legs or knock-knees.

Have You Gained Weight Lately?

Your doctor can see if you are overweight, but he or she should know if the added weight is a recent occurrence or if it has been gradual over the years. If the patient is a child, let the doctor know if there has been a recent spurt in growth.

How Does Your Work or Lifestyle Affect Your Pain?

If you sit all day at a computer, you may develop knee pain as well as low back pain because of lack of exercise. A variety of jobs, sports, and leisure activities may cause or add to people's pain. For example, a surgeon or salesclerk may stand for many hours without a break. A bicycle messenger may develop overuse injury of the knees from pedaling all day. A carpet layer or gardener who kneels for long periods of time could suffer from repetitive strain.

Do You Stay Active and Exercise on a Regular Basis?

Tell your doctor truthfully about the amount of walking and regular exercise you do. Many people who don't exercise say they do because they don't want to appear lazy, but it's important for your doctor to know if you are overdoing a particular exercise, such as running, whether or not you warm up before exercising—or if you haven't been to the gym in months. If knee pain is preventing you from exercising, let the doctor know.

THE INITIAL PHYSICAL EXAMINATION

Once your doctor has obtained your history, the physical examination of your knee is next on the agenda. A clinical examination of your knees should be done while you are standing, sitting, and lying on your back, so the doctor can see any abnormalities in all these positions. For example, if your knees are too close together, or conversely, your legs are bowed, this is best discovered when you are standing. By pressing on your knee with varying degrees of pressure, a doctor can detect increased muscle contraction or spasm. When muscles are at rest, they are soft and pliable. Muscles in spasm, however, are tense, firm to the touch, and may hurt. It is also important to test the flexibility of the hamstrings, quads, and hip muscles. Tightness of these muscles can contribute to knee pain. The flexibility of the iliotibial band should also be checked.

Gait

Watching someone walk can provide a great deal of information about his or her knee pain. If you have an acute ligament injury, you are likely to walk with a limp, a flexed knee, or both in combination. Knee pain can also result from an abnormality in your hip or lower back, which can change the way you walk. It may be helpful to have you step up and down on a short stool to see how you use your knee for climbing and descending stairs. Pain associated with squatting down and standing back up can be helpful in diagnosis.

Range of Motion

Range of motion tests, such as fully extending your knee from a bent position, can tell your doctor a great deal about your knee function. An injured knee may have limited normal motion because of swelling or muscle spasms. If you have difficulty straightening your legs, it may be from tightness of the hamstring or quadriceps muscles, or it can be a result from swelling inside the knee joint. Chronic conditions like arthritis can limit range of motion. Let your doctor know if this limited range is new or old.

Other Tests

There are other specific tests used to help diagnose a knee problem. Bending and rotating the knee may provoke pain or clicking associated with a meniscus tear. The integrity of the four knee ligaments is tested by placing side-to-side stress on the knee to evaluate the MCL and LCL. The integrity of the ACL is tested by flexing the knee at 30-degree and 90-degree angles. The integrity of the PCL is tested by pushing the tibia back with the knee flexed to 90 degrees and comparing the motion to the uninvolved knee.

Your doctor will feel the sides of your kneecap to see if it is painful and may move the kneecap up and down and from side to side to check its flexibility. Your doctor may also raise your leg and push it back toward your chest while you are lying on your back to test your flexibility. If this is done easily, and you feel no discomfort, your muscles are fairly flexible. People with long-term chronic pain or those who are out of condition may be less flexible or will feel tightness or pain more readily when these flexibility tests are performed.

WHAT TO KNOW ABOUT DIAGNOSTIC TESTS

There are scores of diagnostic tests used to identify the cause of disease. Some, like X-rays, are relatively simple and noninvasive. An X-ray of the knee is often done at the time of the initial visit to your doctor to show him the status of the bone and to give him an estimate of the health of the knee joint. An X-ray will diagnose fractures, significant arthritis, and some types of bone tumors, but it does not provide a picture of the soft tissue structures of the knee. Other radiographic tests, such as a CT scan, MRI, and bone scan, help to evaluate these structures and are generally performed in hospitals or radiology centers and require more time and expense.

Always ask your doctor what the diagnostic tests can be expected to determine and how they will help to find the source of pain. Check the reputation of the facility where you are sent for diagnostic tests to ensure that its radiological and diagnostic testing departments are top-notch.

Laboratory Tests

If there is reason to believe the cause of your knee pain may be from a medical condition, then blood tests may be useful. Blood tests may also be performed before you begin a prolonged course of nonsteroidal anti-inflammatory drugs (NSAIDs), which often are prescribed to treat knee pain and inflammation associated with certain knee conditions. These drugs, while effective for knee pain, can cause gastritis, ulcers, loss of kidney function, and liver inflammation. Those who take these drugs for an extended period of time will need their blood, liver function, and kidney function monitored.

CBC (complete blood count) measures red and white blood cells and platelets. A high white blood cell count may be a sign that an infection—such as septic arthritis—is causing the pain. A low red blood cell count, or anemia, may be related to prolonged use of NSAIDs or other medical conditions.

ESR (erythrocyte sedimentation rate) measures the speed at which red blood cells fall in a test tube. An increase in ESR reflects inflammation in the body and may indicate infection, a tumor, or inflammatory arthritis.

CRP (C-reactive protein) is a protein produced by the liver when inflammation is present, and CRP may rise before the ESR becomes elevated. Levels of CRP remain elevated in chronic inflammatory states.

An elevated ESR or CRP calls for additional evaluation in order to determine the medical cause of knee pain.

Other blood and urine tests measure bone chemistry, liver and kidney function, and hormone levels, for example. Conditions such as gout may show an elevated uric acid level in the blood.

Conventional X-rays

X-rays are useful in evaluating the overall appearance of the knee. They provide a way to initially make sure that there is no tumor or fracture, and to check the condition of the growth plate in children's knees. X-rays can diagnose moderate or severe knee arthritis but may not show early arthritis. If an abnormality is seen in an X-ray of a child's knee, it is often necessary to obtain a comparison X-ray of the opposite knee. This is rarely needed in adults.

Keep in mind that few physicians—other than radiologists and orthopedic surgeons—can accurately interpret a musculoskeletal X-ray. This is one more reason to seek out a physician with expertise, even for a routine test like this.

X-rays use ionizing radiation, and it is important to shield areas not being X-rayed from radiation. If you might be pregnant, notify your X-ray technician before any X-ray is taken.

Computed Axial Tomography (CT Scan)

A CT scan, like an MRI, images bone and soft tissue but with less soft tissue detail than an MRI. This test is used to obtain bone detail in conditions such as fractures or tumors involving the knee. A CT scan can be done at many different sites in the body. You lie on your back while a computerized scanner studies a particular area, such as the knee. This test lasts approximately ten to twenty minutes. The radiation dose from a CT scan is considerably higher than a routine X-ray, but it is not considered dangerous if used appropriately.

Magnetic Resonance Imaging (MRI)

Magnetic resonance imaging (MRI) provides images of the body through the use of exposure to a magnetic field without the use of radiation. The strength of the magnet is very important in image quality, so ask your physician to refer you to a high quality facility. Unlike X-rays, MRI can document the status of all of the soft tissue inside and surrounding the knee. It is the most sensitive test for identifying the location of any abnormality and is superior to CT scans in visualizing muscles, ligaments, tendons, and cartilage (articular and meniscal). MRI may be useful in discovering potential sources of knee pain following surgery such as abnormal scar formation.

There are two types of MRI machines: closed MRI and open MRI. The closed MRI produces the best images of the knee, although new open MRI machines can provide reasonable levels of detail. If you get claustrophobic when confined in a closed MRI, find a facility with a staff that can take the time to talk you through the procedure, possibly letting you rest between scanning sequences. A sedative such as Valium and the use of headphones or an eyeshade may help to relax you. An MRI can take from thirty to forty-five minutes, depending on the possible diagnosis.

You cannot have an MRI if you have older metal clips with magnetic properties in your body from prior surgery. There is a risk that the clips will move, or at least heat up, under the influence of the magnet. Most modern clips, made from non-magnetic metals, are safe. If you have any questions, ask your doctor or the staff at the MRI facility. If you have done metal work or welding, you may require a separate test before the MRI to insure that you have no metal fragments in or around your eyes. You cannot have an MRI if you have a pacemaker, as it may affect the ability of the pacemaker to control your cardiac rate and rhythm. If you have metal vascular or cardiac stents, the radiologist will determine if an MRI can be safely performed.

Bone Scan

A bone scan (radionuclide imaging, or nuclear scan) is used to detect stress fractures and abnormalities such as primary bone tumors, infection, and metastatic cancer. Stress fractures are the result of overuse injuries and may not show up on plain X-rays when symptoms are new. When you get an X-ray or a CT scan, the radiation comes from a machine and passes through your body. A nuclear scan works the opposite way: The radiation comes from your body (where it has been injected) and is then detected by a gamma camera. While X-rays can tell you what your knee bones look like, nuclear scans help localize areas of abnormal bone metabolism or activity.

Nuclear scans are safe and painless. A small amount of radioactive material, known as a tracer, is introduced into your body by injection. The camera follows the tracer in the organ or tissue being imaged and records the data on a computer screen. The bone scan is generally done in three phases: two early phases and one delayed phase (three hours post injection), while you are lying on your stomach. Areas reacting to an injury, such as a fracture or inflammation, show up as a dark or "hot" spot on the scan. The increased activity on the scan results from the increased absorption of the radioactive material by the bone cells, which have increased metabolic activity compared with the surrounding cells. The presence of the hot spot does not indicate a specific diagnosis because tumors, infection, fracture, and arthritis can all cause dark spots on the scans. The pattern of increased activity can help the radiologist to create a short list of diagnoses.

A second type of nuclear scan can be done to evaluate the presence of infection. White blood cells are removed from your body, tagged with a radioactive marker, and reinjected. These cells will migrate to the site of infection and can be localized on the scan. Additional radiographic evaluation or blood tests are needed to reach a specific diagnosis.

Nuclear bone scans carry about the same radiation risk as an X-ray. The tracer loses its radioactivity in a few hours, and the material passes out of your body within a day. The only people who should not get such a scan are pregnant women.

Ultrasound

Diagnostic ultrasound can be used to evaluate soft tissue injury such as tendinosis or bursitis and can also be used to guide aspiration or injection near those injuries. Ultrasound sends out high-frequency sound waves that reflect off body structures to create a picture. There is no radiation exposure with this test. The physician or a technician scans your knee with a handheld transducer, or probe, that converts the sound waves that bounce off your body into images on a screen.

Arthrocentesis

Arthrocentesis is a simple procedure that can be performed in your doctor's office. Your doctor will insert a needle into your swollen joint and drain the fluid out of your knee. First, though, he or she may inject the skin with a small amount of local anesthetic such as lidocaine (like the dentist uses) or use a cold spray called ethyl chloride to numb your skin.

The appearance of the fluid can assist your doctor in making a diagnosis. Blood in the fluid may indicate a ligament injury. Blood with fatty droplets in it may indicate an intra-articular fracture. Clear yellow fluid is often seen with meniscal tears, cartilage injuries, and osteoarthritis. Cloudy yellow fluid can result from gout, pseudogout, inflammatory arthritis, or infection.

KEY POINTS

- A physical examination by your physician, a thorough history, and your description of your knee pain are critical in making a diagnosis and developing a plan for treatment.
- Conventional X-rays are routinely performed in the initial evaluation of knee pain.
- MRI scans provide the best demonstration of the soft tissue anatomy inside and outside the knee.
- Blood tests may help determine if your pain has a medical cause and also if long-term use of aspirin or other medications have caused other physical problems.
- Always get the best possible diagnostic tests. Quality varies a great deal, so it may be in your best interests to pay out of pocket for high-quality radiographic tests such as MRIs.
- Ask your doctor what the tests will show and why they are needed.

PART II

TREATING THE CAUSES OF ACUTE AND CHRONIC KNEE PAIN

Chapter 8

Treating Acute Knee Pain from Traumatic Injuries

Torn cartilage, sprained ligaments, tendon ruptures, and knee fractures are the types of injuries that can result from falls, collisions, or twisting accidents. Trauma to your knee can also damage nerves and result in numbness or tingling in your calf or foot. A minor injury may get better with rest, ice to control swelling, and anti-inflammatory medication for pain, but don't ignore a knee injury, because it may be more serious than you think. Most significant knee injuries do require medical attention and, at the very least, a proper diagnosis.

This chapter provides an overview of diagnosis and treatment of traumatic knee injuries. More comprehensive detail on diagnostic tests, treatment procedures, and rehabilitation is provided in other sections of the book. Diagnosis and treatment for overuse injury caused by repetitive action, rather than trauma, are covered in the next chapter.

LIGAMENT INJURIES

As described in chapter 5, ligament injuries frequently occur when you are playing contact sports, or if you pivot your body while your foot is planted in one place. They can also occur from slipping and falling. The ACL and MCL are the most frequently injured. Depending on the grade of the injury (see below), ligament injuries can be treated conservatively or with surgical reconstruction. Sometimes, in a complex injury, more than one ligament must be repaired along with other structures of the knee.

Diagnosing a Ligament Injury

Because ligaments support your knee, when one or more are sprained or torn, your knee will be "loose." Your doctor will examine your knee for such looseness (laxity) while asking you to bend and stretch your knee in various ways. A thorough physical examination of your knee will include several tests to see if your knee stays in the proper position when pressure is applied from different directions. The direction of knee laxity will help your doctor to determine what ligament or ligaments are injured. He or she will see if the tibia shifts forward (ACL), backward (PCL), or side to side (MCL or LCL). An X-ray of your knee will help determine if you have an injury to the bones, but an MRI is frequently needed to determine the extent of a ligament injury. There is often visible bruising with an acute injury.

Ligament injuries are described in three grades from mild to severe:

- **Grade 1** is a first-degree (mild) sprain. There is local pain and swelling but no significant instability. This is a microscopic mild tear in the collagen fibers of the ligament, but full integrity of the ligament is maintained.
- **Grade 2** is a second-degree (moderate) sprain with pain, swelling, and some instability, such as a sense of increased looseness in the knee. This may cause your knee to give way or buckle, particularly with jumping, side motion, or pivoting. This indicates a more substantial tear of collagen fibers, with some loss of continuity of the ligament.
- **Grade 3** is a third-degree (severe) sprain with swelling and marked instability. This kind of sprain disrupts the ligament completely and will not permit your knee to function properly.

Conservative Treatment

As soon as a ligament injury occurs, you should apply ice to control swelling and elevate your knee until you can see a physician. If your ligament is a grade 1 or 2 injury, conservative treatment is often effective, particularly in MCL injury. Your doctor will advise you to rest your knee to give the ligament time to heal and may prescribe a course of physical therapy. Apply ice two or three times a day for fifteen to twenty minutes each time while elevating your knee whenever possible. A bandage or brace may be prescribed to compress the knee and limit swelling. A grade 1 injury is sometimes treated with a light brace or neoprene sleeve (an elastic-like support). A grade 2 or 3 injury is treated with a hinged brace to prevent further injury and protect the healing ligament for four to six weeks.

If your knee is relatively stable, muscle strengthening exercises and anti-inflammatory medication for pain may be all you need. A course of rehabilitation exercises will promote good healing and restore normal walking and range of motion. (See chapter 13 about physical therapy and chapter 18 about conditioning.) Physical therapy is an important part of your treatment plan and may help you avoid surgery; or may, in some cases, help prepare you for surgery and a better recovery.

Treatment with Surgery

The decision to proceed with conservative (nonsurgical) versus surgical treatment for an ACL tear depends on a number of factors. When your doctor discusses the treatment options for a partially or completely torn ACL with you, he or she needs to consider the extent of your knee instability, your age, your activity level, your knee function, and whether or not you will be able to perform the physical therapy needed to recover from surgery.

The ACL is the most commonly reconstructed ligament, but you may also need surgery to repair or reconstruct another if you have injured more than one ligament.

If there is a complete, or high-grade partial tear, and your knee is unstable, then surgery is generally recommended. Because the ACL does not usually heal, it needs to be reconstructed to restore stability to your knee. The torn ACL remnant is removed, and a graft is used to reconstruct the ligament. This graft can be taken either from your own tissue (autograft) or from a tissue bank (allograft). This reconstruction is done with arthroscopic surgery and a small incision for harvesting the tendon to be used as a graft. A strip of tendon from your own patellar or hamstring tendon is passed across the tibia, through the inside of the joint, and secured to both your femur and tibia. It is also possible to use a portion of the quadriceps tendon, but this is a less common graft choice.

The most important factor to consider is whether or not your knee is stable. Does it buckle or give way easily? If you enjoy cutting-and-pivoting sports, an ACL reconstruction is often needed. If you have instability during daily activities, you may also need an ACL reconstruction. The younger you are, the more likely it is that you will need an ACL reconstruction. Here are some examples of ACL injuries occurring at different ages:

> Barbara, fourteen, is a competitive soccer player who plays sports year-round and also enjoys dancing. During a soccer game, she turned to shoot the ball while off balance. Her knee buckled beneath her and she heard a loud pop. When she tried to stand, her knee buckled again. Barbara needed ACL reconstruction because she wanted to continue her sports program. However, most teenagers need ACL reconstruction even if they don't compete in sports, because it is more difficult for them to modify their lifestyle.
>
> Paul, thirty, is of average weight and height, but does no exercise on a regular basis. He tore his ACL while playing football at a high school reunion. An MRI showed a partial tear in his ACL, and he responded well to physical therapy. He had no knee instability with any activity. In fact, six months after his injury, his knee felt perfectly normal. When examined, it became clear that

his ACL injury was not causing any symptoms and was not interfering with his activity level.

Jake, forty-five, tore his ACL while playing in his twice-weekly recreational basketball league. He has young children and wanted to continue his active lifestyle, which also includes running, skiing, and soccer coaching. Although Jake had no instability with daily activities, he did not want to wear a brace and therefore chose ACL reconstruction.

Laura, sixty, skis thirty to forty days a year. She tore her ACL skiing at the end of a long day in icy conditions. Her knee was not unstable with everyday activities, but she wanted to continue to ski vigorously. Laura was initially treated with an ACL brace for skiing but felt her knee slip whenever she curved her body into turns. Twenty years ago, she would not have been a candidate for ACL reconstruction surgery. Now, however, surgery was an option provided that she was medically healthy and prepared to complete the postoperative physical therapy.

Because PCL tears do not result in functional instability as often, they typically can be treated with ice, rest, and rehabilitation. However, if the PCL injury causes significant instability, surgery is needed to repair or reconstruct the ligament. This is similar to ACL reconstruction. Knee function after this surgery is often quite good, although it remains difficult to restore normal function to the PCL. Surgical procedures for the PCL are evolving and improving. Many athletes return to activity without significant impairment after completing a program of rehabilitation.

If your MCL is completely torn or torn in such a way that ligament fibers cannot heal, you may also need surgery. This is quite rare, but when it occurs, it is usually in combination with an ACL or PCL injury, so surgery is required to repair or reconstruct both ligaments. MCL repair or reconstruction is done via open surgery. There are multiple techniques, including primary repair and augmentation with grafted hamstring tendon tissue; or, when laxity is more chronic, reconstruction with allograft tissue. Extended physical rehabilitation (six to nine months) is needed to help people resume their previous levels of activity. A multiligament knee reconstruction is more complex and has an increased risk of postoperative stiffness. Although you may be able to resume full activity, the knee is unlikely to be "perfectly normal" after an injury of this magnitude. (See chapter 15 about surgery.)

Rehabilitation for Ligament Injuries

You will find comprehensive information about rehabilitation and conditioning in chapter 18, but, briefly, a program following ligament injury may include:

- Wearing a brace to control joint movement.
- Active and passive range-of motion exercises to restore flexibility.
- Exercises to strengthen the quadriceps, hamstrings, and hip and calf muscles, as well as to provide muscle strength and support to the knee when weight is placed on it.
- Exercises on a bike or an elliptical trainer to promote recovery of range of motion and strength.
- Use of a CPM (continuous passive motion) machine with a multiligament knee surgery.

Prevention

Many ACL injury-prevention programs for athletes have been developed to assist coaches in designing warm-up and training programs. Two training programs can be found at www.sportsmetrics.net and www.aclprevent.com. These programs appear promising, with some available data demonstrating a decrease in female athletes' risk of injury. No one is yet certain what the ideal components of an ACL injury prevention program should be, but extensive research is ongoing in this area.

Physical therapists can evaluate an athlete's body positioning during activities like squatting, jumping, or changing direction. They can train an athlete utilizing targeted strength training exercises and by incorporating activities involved in his or her sport, for example: throwing or catching using a balance board, and hopping in various patterns. Quality of movement, not quantity, is most important. The goal of this training is to develop healthy movement patterns so they become a habit, and athletes are able to practice a play without thinking about it.

Once you strengthen your muscles, even if you are not an athlete, you can learn movement patterns that will decrease your risk of ligament injuries.

TENDON INJURIES

Conservative treatment may heal a tendon if it is not completely ruptured. However, if surgery is required to repair a torn tendon, it cannot be done arthroscopically because these thick, fibrous cords that attach muscles to bone are outside of the knee joint.

Diagnosis

If there isn't too much swelling around your knee, your doctor may be able to feel a defect in the tendon at the site of the tear and subsequently confirm the extent and location of the tear with MRI. If there is a complete quadriceps tendon tear, your kneecap position will be lower than normal because the quadriceps tendon is no longer attached and can't pull the patella upward. With a complete patellar tendon tear, the patella will sit higher and move upward when the quadriceps contracts, because the attachment to the tibia is disrupted. This change in position of the patella can be seen on a routine lateral X-ray (side view), which helps with diagnosis. In addition, with a complete patellar tendon tear, you will not be able to fully straighten your knee. With a quadriceps tendon tear, you may still be able to extend your knee, but usually you cannot get it completely straight. This is called an extensor lag.

Treatment

If the quadriceps or patellar tendon is completely ruptured, the tendon must be repaired with open surgery. (The patellar tendon cannot be repaired with arthroscopy because this structure is outside of the knee joint: thus, open surgery is required.) An incision is made in the front of the knee to gain access to the tendon. The surgeon will inspect the joint beneath the tendon for other damage while repairing the tendon ends. This may be done as an ambulatory procedure or require an overnight hospital stay, depending on your age and the complexity of the tear. A long leg brace is worn following surgery for six to eight weeks. (See chapter 15 about surgery.)

Rehabilitation

After surgical repair of a partial or complete tendon tear, you will need to follow a rehabilitation program that is designed specifically for your injury. The exercises help to restore your ability to bend and straighten your knee and to restore full mobility to your kneecap and patellofemoral joint. Six to nine months of rehabilitation may be needed after tendon surgery, although you can return to many activities, such as walking, within eight to twelve weeks.

Prevention

The best way to prevent injuries to the tendons is to keep the muscles that support those tendons strong and flexible. Stretching and strengthening exercises will help prevent tendon injuries, or make them less likely.

MENISCUS INJURIES

Your age will be a consideration in how your meniscus injury is treated. For example, if you are over forty and have a degenerative meniscus tear, your cartilage may be injured because of a mild trauma, such as taking a wrong step. If the tear is small, it's possible that physical therapy is all that you need. If you are younger, and your meniscus was torn because of considerable trauma, there's a higher probability that you will need surgery.

Diagnosis

The diagnosis of a meniscus injury is based on history, physical exam, and imaging studies. Once your doctor has listened to your description of how the pain and swelling began and conducted a physical exam, X-rays and an MRI may be recommended to confirm the diagnosis.

Treatment

If your meniscus tear is of the degenerative type, your doctor may recommend physical therapy to help restore your range of motion and strength, and NSAIDs to ease inflammation and pain. Exercises designed to build up your quadriceps and hamstrings and increase your flexibility and strength, such as riding a stationary bike or exercising in a pool, may be helpful.

If your meniscus injury is more severe or is the result of significant trauma and does not respond to conservative treatment, arthroscopic surgery may be needed to remove or repair the tear. The best results of surgical treatment for a meniscus injury are obtained if there is no damage to the articular cartilage and if you have an intact ACL. If you do not have an intact ACL, you are at risk for repeat meniscus tears or failure of meniscus repair because of the knee's rotational instability.

The decision whether to repair the meniscus or to remove the torn piece depends on your age and the complexity of the tear. Repair is uncommon for anyone over forty.

The location of the meniscus tear is important because the fibrocartilage has a blood supply that extends from the periphery to about one-third of the way into the meniscus. Tears in this vascular zone (meaning where there is blood flow) are called "red-red" tears because the blood supply to both sides of the tear help it repair quickly. "Red-white" tears in the middle of the meniscus may be repaired, but the surgery may be less successful because blood supply is present on only one side of the tear. Tears in the inner third of the meniscus, or "white-white" tears, are generally removed. If repair is attempted on a white-white tear, special techniques are used to improve the healing response of this tissue.

Rehabilitation

Recovery time following meniscus surgery depends on whether the meniscus has been repaired or removed. Removal of a small meniscus tear has a good prognosis, and you can generally return to full activity, including sports, in four to eight weeks. The timing of your return to sports depends on recovery of full range of motion and strength and the absence of pain and swelling. Some people respond very quickly following meniscus surgery, while others have a slower recovery from an identical surgical procedure.

Recovery following meniscus repair is slower, as activity for the first six weeks is limited, and bracing is often used. It is necessary to protect the repair site while the tear heals. The timing of your return to sports, weight-bearing status, and use of a postoperative brace depends on your age; the size, type, and location of the tear; and the stability of the repair. It may take four to six months to return to full activity after a meniscus repair.

Prevention

To lower your risk for further injury of your meniscus, your doctor may recommend special exercises designed to build up your quadriceps and hamstrings, and increase your flexibility and strength:

- Ride a stationary bicycle to warm up your knee before straightening and raising your leg.
- Extend your leg while sitting (a weight may be worn on the ankle).
- Raise your leg while lying on your stomach.
- Exercise in a pool by walking as fast as possible in chest-deep water; perform small flutter kicks while holding on to the side of the pool; and raise each leg 90 degrees in chest-deep water while pressing your back against the side of the pool.

Before beginning any type of exercise program, consult your doctor or physical therapist to learn which exercises are appropriate for you and how to do them correctly. (See chapter 18 on conditioning.)

OSTEOCHONDRITIS DISSECANS (OCD)

Treatment of OCD will depend on age. For example, if OCD is diagnosed in a child with open growth plates, it may be possible to treat it conservatively to permit healing of the fragment. If the fragment of cartilage and bone is beginning to separate from the end of the femur, or if there is a loose fragment of bone or cartilage in the knee joint, then surgery is required. (See chapter 4 for a complete description of this condition.)

Diagnosis

An X-ray will show the area of bone abnormality and will prompt additional evaluation. An MRI can determine the condition of the overlying cartilage and the bone fragment in OCD. In the early stages, the bone and cartilage are intact, with no separation from the bone. In the middle stage, a thin line of fluid will separate the OCD from its "bed" on the femur. In the later stages of the disease, the fragment may form a "trapdoor" type of flap or may float free within the joint. These characteristics can be clearly defined on MRI.

Treatment

In a young person with open growth plates, OCD can initially be treated with a knee brace or cast to restrict range of motion and crutches to restrict weight bearing. If the fragment is separated from the bone but not completely detached, an arthroscopic procedure is indicated. Pins or screws can be surgically inserted into the cartilage and bone fragment to repair the fragment and fix it in place. It is also necessary to stimulate a new blood supply at the time of repair to help the bone fragments heal to the underlying bone. If the fragments are loose, the surgeon may remove them from the knee or may add bone graft and fix the fragments in position. Fragments that cannot be repaired are removed, and the cavity is drilled or scraped to stimulate the growth of a scarlike cartilage replacement. If a large fragment is removed, your surgeon may take a plug of cartilage and bone from another site in your knee and place it in the cavity. (See chapter 15 about surgery.)

Rehabilitation

A follow-up program of physical therapy is usually necessary to return to full strength and stability of the knee. Recovery from any of these surgical procedures will require a period of time on crutches, and you may need a brace and use of a CPM machine.

Prevention

Unfortunately, the cause of OCD in the knee remains uncertain, so we do not know how to prevent this lesion. However, early diagnosis of OCD can improve the response to both conservative and surgical treatments. If a child, adolescent, or young adult develops knee pain in the absence of trauma, a visit to the orthopedic surgeon is indicated to obtain a clear diagnosis.

PATELLAR SUBLUXATION AND DISLOCATION

When your kneecap subluxes (patellar subluxation) or does not track properly in the trochlear groove, there are several ways to treat it, depending on the cause. When the patella dislocates, surgery is often required. (For information about patellar subluxation and dislocation, see chapter 4.)

Treatment

The initial treatment for patellar subluxation is conservative. Bracing and taping will help to control the motion of your kneecap, and physical therapy will help to strengthen your quadriceps and achieve balance of the soft tissues necessary to keep your patella centered in the trochlear groove. Better footwear may also be suggested as a way to control gait and knee position, which may reduce pressure on your kneecap if you are a runner. A supportive shoe can help with knee alignment.

If conservative therapy doesn't work, surgery may be necessary, especially if there is significant pain or recurrent dislocation. A minimum of six months of conservative treatment is generally indicated prior to proceeding with patellofemoral surgery (in the absence of significant trauma), as many patients respond to conservative treatment. A preoperative MRI will assess the status of the articular cartilage surfaces and can provide your surgeon with information about the status of the retinaculum and supporting structures. By looking into the knee with an arthroscopic camera, the orthopedic surgeon can see what is needed to correct the alignment of the knee in the groove. There can be excessive lateral tension pulling the patella laterally or causing patellar tilt. This, combined with lax medial support ligaments, increases the risk of patellar subluxation.

Patellofemoral surgery is done with arthroscopic, open, and combined approaches. If the supporting structures on the outside of your knee are tight and those on the inside are too loose, then a combination of lateral release and medial repair is done. The lateral release cuts the tight lateral retinaculum, a supporting ligamentlike structure, so the kneecap can move in toward the middle of the groove. Then your surgeon may rebuild the ligament known as the medial patellofemoral ligament (MPFL), which holds the kneecap in place; or she may tighten the medial retinaculum. If your kneecap dislocation has been caused by trauma, and the MPFL is torn, a primary repair of the MPFL may be possible.

Some people dislocate their kneecaps because of the misalignment of their thigh, knee, and shin. This problem requires a distal realignment, which changes the position of the bony attachment of the patellar tendon to stabilize or unload the patella. Open patellofemoral surgery can also be performed to alter the forces on an arthritic patella.

Rehabilitation

Open patellofemoral surgery requires four to six weeks of a long leg brace and the use of crutches for a variable period of time. Six months of postoperative physical therapy may be needed to restore full range of motion and strength.

Prevention

If you know you are loose jointed, you should work with your doctor or physical therapist to develop a plan of therapy to prevent possible future episodes of subluxation or dislocation.

PATELLA FRACTURE

Martin, fifty years old and well over six feet tall, was sitting next to the driver in a small car that was involved in a traffic accident. Although he was wearing a seat belt, the force of the collision pushed the dashboard into the lower part of his kneecaps. Both were broken. X-rays taken in the emergency room demonstrated a displaced fracture of one patella and a hairline fracture, or crack, of the other. One knee required open reduction internal fixation (ORIF) of the fragments, and the other knee was treated with a long leg brace. ORIF is a method of repairing and stabilizing the fractured bone with plates and screws and sometimes a metal wire.

When you fracture your patella, you may hear a crack or pop, and you are likely to suffer severe pain and swelling at the site of a fracture. It will be difficult to extend or bend your knee. Patella fractures come in all degrees of complexity. A crack in bone may cause only moderate pain, while an open fracture with exposed bone is a surgical emergency. If the bone shatters into fragments, it may distort your normal knee contours.

Diagnosis

A patellar fracture requires emergency medical treatment to determine the extent of injury and necessary treatment. X-rays are taken to see the complexity of the fracture. The emergency room physician may ask you to try a straight leg raise to test the function of your quadriceps tendon and its attachment to your patella. Any disruption of the quadriceps tendon, patella, or patellar tendon can prevent you from raising your leg. If you can perform a straight leg raise, and the bone fragments are not displaced or separated, then it may be possible to treat your fracture without surgery.

Treatment

If pieces of bone are not displaced, you may be treated in a cast or brace to immobilize the patella and allow the bone to heal.

Surgery is needed when the patella is in multiple fragments, or if fragments have moved from their original positions. An incision is made over the front of your knee, and the pieces of bone are repaired using a combination of wire, sutures, and metal pins or screws.

Your leg will generally be placed in a well-padded splint immediately following surgery and subsequently in a cast or long leg brace, depending on the stability of the repair. Pain medication, rest, ice, and elevation will be prescribed. You will need crutches or a cane for walking. If there has been significant injury to the articular cartilage, and the fracture repair is stable, your surgeon may recommend the use of a CPM machine to facilitate healing of the cartilage surface. While your leg is immobilized, it's important to try to maintain your strength by exercising muscles that are not immobilized, as directed by your surgeon. For example, your intact leg will support more of your weight, and your arms and shoulders will need strength to get around with crutches. Always follow your surgeon's recommendations, which are guided by the type of fracture and the stability of the repair.

Rehabilitation

Once the cast or brace is removed after surgery, you will need to periodically apply ice packs to the area to help ease the pain. Once it is safe to do so, your surgeon will prescribe physical therapy that may include ice, heat, ultrasound, electric stimulation, massage, and a program of therapeutic exercises. The timing of these exercises depends on the type of repair done and the extent of fracture healing. The fracture is not considered fully healed until follow-up X-rays show complete bone union. The average healing time for a patellar fracture ranges from six to twelve weeks, with a gradual resumption of walking and bending. However, this may take longer if you resume some activities (such as deep bending) too soon. Even after healing, you may be prone to future knee problems. This is common if there has been injury to or loss of cartilage from the articular surface of the kneecap at the time of the fracture. You might also develop posttraumatic arthritis as a result of the initial trauma to your knee.

If you develop increased pain, fever, or redness after surgery, or notice swelling in your foot and calf, you may have an infection or a blood clot in your calf. You should contact your surgeon immediately. Other complications that require your physician's immediate attention are headache, muscle aches, nausea, vomiting, or loss of feeling.

Prevention

While you can't always avoid accidents, two things you can do to prevent knee fracture is to maintain a healthy weight and always wear a seat belt in a car. Being overweight and hitting the dashboard with your knees are the biggest causes of knee fracture.

KEY POINTS

- Conservative treatment with ice, rest, bracing, and strengthening exercises may be all you need with a mild ligament sprain, but always see a doctor if the pain doesn't stop within a few days.
- A torn ligament will not heal and may need to be reconstructed with a graft from your own body or a tissue bank, but surgery depends on your age, activity level, and general health.
- Mild tendon injuries are generally treated conservatively. However, if the tendon is ruptured, open surgery is required to repair it because these tendons are outside the area of the knee joint; therefore, arthroscopic surgery is not applicable.
- When conservative treatment doesn't heal a meniscus injury, arthroscopic surgery is required.
- OCD in a child with open growth plates can sometimes be treated conservatively, but in an adult or child the disease may require surgery if there is a loose piece of bone and/or cartilage.
- Patellar subluxation is generally treated with taping or bracing, but current dislocation requires surgery.
- A patella fracture is a medical emergency if it is an open fracture with exposed bone or the bone is in pieces. If only cracked, it can be fixed with a brace or cast until it heals.

Chapter 9

Treating Chronic Knee Pain
from Overuse Injuries

It would be interesting to know how many Tour de France cyclists develop tendinitis during their grueling multiday ride through the towns and countryside. Perhaps their doctors and trainers keep them in such good shape that it never occurs, but tendinitis, an overuse injury, is more likely to happen to bike enthusiasts who decide to go on a weeklong cycling vacation without any practice or training. An occasional bike ride to the local park will not prepare you for riding eight hours a day through the green hills of Ireland for a week.

Overuse injuries to your knee occur as repetitive motion or positions put continuous stress on your ligaments, tendons, cartilage, and/or bursae. Runners are at risk for pain on the outside of their knees from the continuous friction of the iliotibial band rubbing over the lateral aspect of the knee each time their feet hit the pavement. Little League catchers who kneel for hours at a time can overtax growing bones and muscles around the knee.

As an overuse injury progresses, the pain will generally get worse or begin earlier into the activity. Your knee may swell and feel warm to the touch as inflammation develops. When overuse injuries are caused by a particular activity, there are steps you can take to prevent further injury, such as improving strength and flexibility or using knee pads. But first, you need to find out the cause of the overuse injury, treat it, and refrain from the activity that is causing it until your pain is gone.

BURSITIS

Kneeling on a hard surface for prolonged periods of time is the most common cause of prepatellar bursitis of the knee, which is how it became known as housemaid's knee. The repetitive nature of kneeling irritates and thickens the bursa over time. A good example is Jack from chapter 2, who, in order to keep his flooring business profitable, spent too much time kneeling without using knee pads. Jack developed prepatellar bursitis, which happens to people in his line of work and to gardeners who spend long periods of time kneeling. Three types of bursitis affect the knee. In addition to prepatellar bursitis, there is pes anserine bursitis at the inner side of the knee, and iliotibial band bursitis on the outer side.

Bursae are sacs of fluid located where tendons and muscles move over the bones. (See chapter 1.) While bursitis can occur in other joints, such as shoulders and elbows, it is common in the knee. A direct injury such as a fall or blow to the knee, an infection, or an underlying medical condition such as gout or obesity can result in bursitis, but it is most often caused by overuse.

Prepatellar bursitis affects the front of your knee. You may have pain when you bend or straighten the joint. Your level of activity affects the amount of swelling that occurs. For example, if you kneel for a long period of time, the prepatellar bursa may distend (fill up) with fluid and have the appearance of a small water balloon. Pain, swelling, and redness at the front of your knee are the most frequent symptoms, and there may be small lumps under the skin over your kneecap. These lumps are areas of thickened bursae that have formed because of chronic irritation.

Pes anserine bursitis causes slowly developing pain and tenderness on the inside (medial aspect) of the knee, two to three inches below the joint. Pain also increases with exercise, climbing stairs, or straightening your knee after a period of prolonged bending. The pes anserine bursa is located between the tibia and three tendons (semitendinosus, gracilis, and sartorius) that attach to the inside of the tibia. Runners are particularly susceptible to this form of bursitis when they neglect to stretch their hamstring muscles, if they do excessive downhill running, or if they increase mileage too rapidly. People with osteoarthritis can also develop this type of bursitis, and it appears commonly in middle-aged women. The cause of pes anserine bursitis in these women is unknown, but it may relate to changes in gait, or a weakness of hip and thigh muscles, resulting in overuse of the hamstrings. This may occur as a type of compensation in someone with knee pain from another cause.

Iliotibial bursitis affects the long fibrous structure that runs along the outside of your thigh from hip to knee. This condition, sometimes called iliotibial band friction syndrome, is caused by the ITB rubbing against the bursa on the outside of the end of the femur, just above the knee joint, which causes inflammation. It is a common overuse injury in runners and cyclists. If you run on a sloped surface, or your running shoes are worn out, this may increase your risk for ITB problems. You may feel a sharp, burning pain along the outside of your knee during or after running or cycling. If you continue this activity, you may find it more difficult to straighten your knee because of pain.

Diagnosis

In diagnosing bursitis, your doctor will examine your knee to see where it hurts and will test your flexibility to see if that causes discomfort. Prepatellar bursitis is an easy diagnosis to make, as the bursa is often visibly swollen. If your doctor suspects infection is possible, fluid may be removed from your knee for analysis before determining the best treatment for you. Pes anserine and ITB bursitis may be more difficult to diagnose because of overlapping soft tissue structures. It is important to rule out other possible bony sources of pain with an X-ray. MRI is generally not necessary to make this diagnosis.

Treatment

If this is your first bout with bursitis, the swelling should resolve with activity modification, the use of ice several times a day, and anti-inflammatory medications as directed by your doctor. In some people, a short course of physical therapy can help improve strength, flexibility, and endurance, which will decrease the chance that ITB or pes bursitis will recur. If your bursitis is chronic and does not respond to conservative treatment, your doctor may recommend a cortisone injection (see chapter 14 about medications).

Surgically removing the bursa is rarely needed. If the prepatellar bursa is infected, it will need to be drained (aspirated) with a needle several times before further treatment. During this time, you will need to take antibiotics that are prescribed to treat the specific bacteria causing the infection. (The bacteria are identified when the drained fluid from your bursa is sent to a microbiology laboratory.) If an infection does not respond to medical treatment, open surgery may be necessary to remove the infected bursa to allow the antibiotics to cure the infection.

Rehabilitation

After this procedure, you will need to stay off your feet for several days to allow the knee to heal.

Prevention

A physical therapy program of stretching exercises is important to improve the flexibility of muscles and soft tissue around your knee to help you avoid pes anserine and iliotibial band bursitis by using your muscles more efficiently.

If you cannot completely avoid the provocative activity, relieve the pressure by taking regular breaks. If you must kneel for prolonged periods, as when laying carpet or gardening, use protective cushions or knee pads.

TENDINITIS

Tendinitis is an overuse injury of one or more tendons, the thick, fibrous cords that attach muscle to bone. Runners, skiers, cyclists, jumping athletes, and active people are prone to develop inflammation in the patellar and quadriceps tendons, which connect the quadriceps muscle to the patella and tibia. The quadriceps tendon connects the quad muscle to the knee, and the patellar tendon extends from that tendon, over the knee, and to the tibia.

Tendinitis can occur in one or both knees. Symptoms include pain just below the kneecap (patellar tendinitis) or above the kneecap (quadriceps tendinitis) when you stand up or begin an activity. Pain usually intensifies when you play a sport that involves jumping, such as volleyball or basketball. Patellar tendinitis is sometimes called jumper's knee because the muscle contraction and force of hitting the ground after a jump strain the tendon. The pain may improve as you warm up during play and may worsen after completing the activity. After repeated stress, the tendon may become inflamed, tear, or begin to degenerate (tendinosis). This is most common in jumping and running athletes or workers who lift heavy objects in a repetitive fashion.

Diagnosis

The diagnosis of where the tendinitis is located—at the patellar or quadriceps tendon—is made during your physical exam. Your doctor will find a localized area of pain that may or may not be accompanied by swelling or increased warmth. In cases of chronic tendon pain, an MRI will show the extent of tendon degeneration, scarring, or a partial tear of either tendon. Your physician will also assess your strength and flexibility. Weak and tight muscles may increase your risk of developing tendinitis.

Treatment

Initially, tendinitis is treated with ice, rest, elimination of the provocative activity, and taking NSAIDs such as aspirin or ibuprofen to relieve pain and decrease inflammation and swelling. This is followed by rehabilitation exercise. (For information about torn tendons, see chapter 5.)

Prevention

It is important to be well conditioned when you participate in lengthy or repetitive exercise. Strengthen your quadriceps, hamstring, and calf muscles to help decrease the stress on the tendons. You also need to have good flexibility of your quadriceps, hip flexors, and hamstrings. It may also be helpful to reduce pressure on your tendons by supporting your knee with an elastic knee strap or sleeve (sold in most drugstores). Warm up before exercise to activate your muscles and increase flexibility before putting strain on your tendons. Gradually increase the duration and frequency of exercise, since the most common cause of overuse injury is "too much, too soon."

ILIOTIBIAL BAND (ITB) SYNDROME

The long and strong fibrous band that extends from the outside of your femur, down your thigh, and attaches to the outside of your tibia is the iliotibial band (ITB). This band helps you rotate your hip and move your lower legs. When the ITB becomes very tight and rubs against the outside end of the femur, it can cause a sharp, burning pain and inflammation. You can experience pain along the entire length of the ITB, where it crosses the end of the femur, or where it attaches to the top of the tibia, at a site called Gerdy's tubercle.

In the early stages of ITB syndrome, a leading cause of knee pain in runners, the pain goes away with rest, but with time it may persist when you walk or go up and down stairs. ITB syndrome does not affect the motion of your knee (although it may be hard to straighten your leg fully because of pain), and swelling is rare. The pain in the side of your knee may radiate up the side of your thigh. You may feel a snap or grinding on the outside of your knee when you bend and then straighten it. Running on hard or banked surfaces and wearing worn-out or improper running shoes also contribute to the condition. ITB syndrome is also common in cyclists because that same band rubs the outside of the knee when pedaling. In addition to lack of ITB stretching, the syndrome can be caused by riding a bike with a seat that is too low or foot pedals in the wrong position.

Diagnosis

When you have pain from ITB syndrome, you tend to walk with your knee slightly bent to prevent the ITB from rubbing against it. An Ober's test should be performed so that your physician can determine how tight your ITB is. This exam calls for you to lie on your unaffected side while the doctor determines how tight your ITB is.

Before making treatment plans, your doctor will want to rule out other causes of lateral knee pain such as degenerative joint disease, stress fracture, collateral ligament sprain, meniscus tear, or patellofemoral stress syndrome.

Treatment

Initially, treatment of ITB syndrome is aimed at reducing pain and inflammation with NSAIDs, ice, rest, and gentle stretching. The syndrome usually disappears if you reduce the activity and perform the stretching exercises. However, the ultimate goal of treatment is to minimize the friction of the ITB as it slides over the femur, generally with a program of stretching exercises. Your doctor may recommend a physical therapist trained in treating this condition.

A stretching regimen should also focus on neighboring muscles; specifically, the hamstrings, quadriceps, and hip abductor muscles on the outer thigh. The abductors move the leg away from the body. These muscles can be worked with a variety of side-lying leg lifts. See chapter 18 about conditioning for stretching examples.

If the pain and swelling persist after extensive conservative treatment, your doctor may prescribe a local corticosteroid injection into the bursa to relieve pain and inflammation. In very rare cases, surgery may be necessary to lengthen the ITB so that it isn't stretched too tightly over the bone.

Prevention

Iliotibial band syndrome can be prevented by developing a sensible plan for your sport or job so that you are not overusing the ligament. It is important to allow the surrounding tendons and muscles to rest between bouts of exertion and to always warm up with stretching exercises.

PATELLOFEMORAL PAIN AND CHONDROMALACIA OF THE PATELLA

Patellofemoral pain and chondromalacia of the patella (CMP) are conditions caused by overload, injury, or degeneration of patella articular cartilage. They have similar symptoms, so correct diagnosis is crucial to proper treatment (see chapter 5 about these conditions). The back of your patella is lined with articular cartilage that helps it glide in the trochlear groove when you bend and straighten your knee.

Diagnosis

An X-ray taken with the knee slightly bent may reveal the lateral displacement or tilt of the kneecap. If the space between the patella and the trochlear groove (also called the patellofemoral joint) is narrowed, CMP or early patellofemoral arthritis may be the cause of pain. A side view of the knee may show a high-riding or low-riding patella.

Patellofemoral pain syndrome describes pain at the patellofemoral joint without radiographic or MRI evidence of cartilage breakdown. The diagnosis of chondromalacia, which is softening or mild roughness of the cartilage, is made on MRI or an arthroscopic exam of the cartilage. The MRI is the ideal nonoperative method for evaluating the patellofemoral cartilage. A well done MRI will show cartilage thickness and the presence of articular cartilage softening, roughness, flaps, or localized loss.

Treatment

It is extremely important to avoid activities that cause pain in your knee, so that you don't prolong your recovery time. For example, if the leg extension machine at your gym causes your knee to hurt, don't use it. See if there is an arc of motion that does not cause pain. There are also other ways to strengthen your quads without causing further pain and injury. Your doctor may prescribe physical therapy or a home exercise program to help you improve the strength and flexibility of critical muscles and structures around your knee. Swimming, riding a stationary bike, or using a cross-country ski machine or elliptical trainer can provide good cardiovascular conditioning for people with this condition. (See chapter 18 on conditioning.)

In most cases, the symptoms of chondromalacia are treated by discontinuing the activity that is causing symptoms, taking pain medication, and doing exercises to strengthen the knee and improve flexibility. Once the cartilage has been damaged, there is nothing that can be done to restore a normal surface.

In many cases, physical therapy can be specifically targeted to the cause of your patellofemoral pain. Your therapist may employ a technique called patellar taping to assist in balancing the patella while strength and flexibility improve.

Electrical stimulation and biofeedback (see chapters 13 and 17 respectively), may also be used to help you strengthen the muscles. (See chapter 13 about physical therapy.)

If you need to stay active in sports, a knee brace may help stabilize your kneecap. Patellofemoral braces come in many designs of different complexity. The most common brace is a neoprene sleeve with a cutout for the kneecap and a horse-shoe-shaped pad based laterally. This helps to center the patella in the trochlea and keep your kneecap from tracking laterally. (See chapter 12 about knee bracing.)

If these treatments don't improve your symptoms, and you have more severe damage to your patellofemoral carti-lage, your surgeon may recommend arthroscopic surgery to smooth the surface of the cartilage and to remove car-tilage fragments that can cause catching or the sense of locking during bending and straightening. In more severe cases, surgery may be necessary to correct the angle of the kneecap, to unload areas of cartilage wear, or to reposition parts that are out of alignment. One procedure performed to correct patellar tilt is a lateral release. The tight lateral retinaculum is cut to allow the patella to resume a more normal position. Thin scar tissue eventually fills in the gap created by the surgery. This surgery takes thirty to forty-five minutes and is performed arthroscopically under regional or general anesthesia. A few days on crutches and plenty of rest will help to speed your recovery. Then you can gradu-ally resume normal activities—with your doctor's advice. (See chapter 15 about surgery.) The indications for lateral release are very specific, and this procedure should be per-formed to correct patellar tilt only.

If cartilage loss is severe but localized, there are new tech-niques being developed for cartilage resurfacing. Increasingly, doctors are using osteochondral grafting, in which a plug of bone and healthy cartilage is harvested from one area and transplanted to the injury site.

Another relatively new technique is known as autologous chondrocyte implantation, or ACI. It involves harvesting healthy cartilage cells, cultivating them in a lab, and implanting them under a patch at the site of cartilage loss.

Prevention

You don't need to stop all activities, but you should limit or avoid particular activities or movements that aggravate your condition. If you are a runner, reduce your mileage and avoid steps, hills, and uneven surfaces, which may exacerbate pain. Try lower-impact activities, such as walking, until the pain subsides. Apply ice several times a day and after workouts. Buy new athletic shoes with good arch support and cushioning. Look for sports shoes that are specific for the activity that you do. Don't run in basketball sneakers, and don't play basketball in track shoes.

OSGOOD-SCHLATTER DISEASE

Osgood-Schlatter disease is an overuse injury that develops during a child's growth years to cause knee pain. The symptoms generally resolve when a child stops growing because of closure of the tibial apophysis (growth plate), and the pain and swelling go away. In some susceptible teenagers, symptoms may last two to three years.

Diagnosis

A clinical exam can diagnose the presence of Osgood-Schlatter disease, but X-rays of the knee are important to determine the severity of the disease and to eliminate other sources of adolescent knee pain such as osteomyelitis (bone infection) and bone tumor. Your doctor should be able to see the prominence of the tibial tubercle, a bone growth extending from the top of the shin. The distal patellar tendon and soft tissue may also be tender.

The X-ray will show widening or fragmentation of the apophyseal growth plate. The degree of widening on the X-ray will help guide your doctor to determine any activity limitations or restrictions. In a growing child, a thorough hip exam should be part of any knee evaluation because hip problems can often refer pain to the knee, so don't be surprised when your physician also examines your child's hip.

Treatment

Osgood-Schlatter disease usually resolves with avoidance of the provocative activity and the application of ice. Stretching and strengthening exercises may help. Your doctor may limit participation in vigorous sports, particularly if there is significant widening or fragmentation of the tibial apophysis. If the symptoms are less severe, children who wish to continue moderate or less stressful sports may need to wear knee pads for protection and apply ice to the knee after the activity.

The goal of treatment is to reduce pain and swelling with the use of ice and stretching. Anti-inflammatory medications, even over-the-counter medications such as Aleve and Motrin, should not be given to children on a regular basis unless discussed with your pediatrician. If weakness and pain get worse with activity, the treatment may require rest for several months, followed by a conditioning program.

Prevention

Excess kneeling and squatting should be avoided. If your child is a Little League catcher, perhaps he or she should play a position that does not require squatting. Avoiding activities such as jumping rope, basketball, and sprinting if they cause knee pain may be helpful. Stretching the quadriceps and hamstring muscles is important, particularly during adolescence, when children have significant growth spurts. Cutting back on activities may distress a child who plays at a competitive level, so it is important to reassure him or her that the condition will ultimately resolve.

KEY POINTS

- Bursitis is generally treated by avoiding the activity that causes the problem and taking NSAIDs for pain relief.
- Tendinitis can be treated conservatively with icing and rest as well as rehabilitative physical therapy.
- Iliotibial band syndrome is also treated with rest, icing, and gentle stretching.

- Patellofemoral pain and chondromalacia of the patella can be treated with bracing and rehabilitation, but if severe, arthroscopic surgery to resurface the knee cartilage may be necessary.
- Osgood-Schlatter disease is treated by avoiding the activity that aggravates it, along with rest, icing, elevating, and conditioning with stretching and strengthening exercises.

Chapter 10

Treating Chronic Knee Pain from Arthritis and Other Inflammatory Conditions

When a car is no longer driven every day but allowed to sit in the garage and rust, it may not operate as efficiently as it once did. It may sputter and moan when you start it. It may cough out unhealthy exhaust. But if the car is cared for, given regular repairs and oil changes, and is taken out for a ride every day, it will probably run well for a long time. The same goes for people who suffer from arthritis in their knees. As knee cartilage degenerates and causes pain when you walk or bend your knees, you need to pamper your knees. Proper medical treatment and continued appropriate use are the first lines of therapy for arthritis and other inflammatory knee conditions.

Arthritis means joint inflammation and refers to a group of diseases that cause pain, swelling, stiffness, and loss of motion in the joints. When your knee is damaged as a result of a traumatic injury, an infection, an autoimmune condition, or the process of cartilage aging and degeneration, the result is one of a number of types of arthritis: post-traumatic, septic, inflammatory, or osteoarthritis. In septic or inflammatory arthritis, a series of events is triggered in your body. Specialized sentinel cells stationed throughout your body alert your immune system that bacteria may be present or something is amiss. Some of these cells—mast cells—release histamine, a chemical that makes nearby small blood vessels (capillaries) leaky so that small amounts of plasma and cells can pour out and slow down the invading bacteria. At the same time, macrophages, another group of sentinel cells, begin an immediate counterattack by releasing cytokines—chemicals that signal for reinforcements. Soon your injured knee is flooded with immune cells that destroy pathogens and damaged tissue alike. In this war, both sides are wiped out. Your knee is literally at war with itself. As a result, it swells, feels hot, hurts, and does not function properly.

Treatment for inflammatory arthritis varies according to the specific type, but most aim to control pain and swelling, to prevent the condition from getting worse, and to limit the effect of the arthritis on your daily life. For each type of inflammatory arthritis, the diagnosis and treatment are explained here, but at the end of the chapter you will find some tips for lifestyle changes that may help reduce pain for all types of arthritis. Most arthritis is not curable, but symptoms can be managed. Some types, such as rheumatoid arthritis, go through periods of remission and flares, but most arthritis symptoms are treatable, and with modern medications, the disease progress can be modified and slowed.

OSTEOARTHRITIS

The most common type of arthritis is osteoarthritis (see chapter 5), which affects older people and women more frequently than men. It is a degenerative disease of the articular cartilage that results in progressive thinning and ultimate loss of the gliding surface. Osteoarthritis usually develops slowly over a period of time, and the degree of pain, swelling, and functional disability varies. In the early stages of osteoarthritis, some localized soreness when you run, jump, or put a heavy load on your knee may be all you feel. But as time progresses and the degeneration causes knee inflammation, you may experience pain even after you have stopped the activity. Eventually you may have pain with walking, climbing stairs, sitting for prolonged periods, or even just standing.

Diagnosis

In addition to a comprehensive physical examination, X-ray is the primary diagnostic test for osteoarthritis. While an X-ray does not show the cartilage or meniscus, it does show the space between the bones filled by those soft tissues. Mild arthritis may appear normal or show a subtle narrowing of the joint space between the femur and tibia or between the patella and femur. Osteophytes, which are small spurs of bone that form at the edge of the degenerating joint, can also be detected on an X-ray.

If the subtle cartilage loss of early arthritis cannot be detected on an X-ray, you need an MRI to evaluate the meniscus and articular cartilage. Often, early osteoarthritis is found through an MRI performed to evaluate a meniscus or ligament injury in someone with a history of osteoarthritis symptoms. Moderate or severe arthritis can be diagnosed with X-rays alone. In severe arthritis, the femur and tibia, or the femur and patella, will appear to be touching. For an accurate assessment of the degree of arthritis, it is important that the X-ray be taken while you are bearing weight. X-rays taken while the patient is lying down can overestimate joint space because of lack of load on the joint.

Treatment

Treatment for osteoarthritis depends on your age, general health, and desired activity level. If your condition is mild, conservative treatment consisting of rest, ice, physical therapy, and intermittent use of over-the-counter medications such as ibuprofen (Motrin) or acetaminophen (Tylenol) may suffice.

A popular oral supplement for treating the symptoms of osteoarthritis is a mixture of glucosamine and chondroitin sulfate, compounds that are naturally manufactured by the body. Supplements don't work for everyone, and you should never take them without consulting your doctor. Medical treatment combined with lifestyle changes, such as regular exercise, weight loss, and avoiding provocative activity are used to manage your arthritis. For example, if you are an avid runner who is developing osteoarthritis, your doctor may recommend decreasing your mileage, cross training on a bike or elliptical trainer, or running fewer days a week.

For more intense pain or an acute flare of osteoarthritis,

your doctor may prescribe stronger anti-inflammatory medication or a viscosupplementation injection to improve lubrication in the joint (see chapter 14).

Arthroscopic surgery (arthroscopy) is sometimes indicated in people with mild or moderate osteoarthritis when there is also a symptomatic meniscus tear. If your knee is malaligned because of localized moderate arthritis, you may be treated with an osteotomy to realign the knee and unload the symptomatic compartment (see chapter 15 about surgery). There are braces available that can unload the medial or lateral compartment of the knee. These can also be used to manage arthritis pain and can be very effective. When severe, osteoarthritis can be treated surgically with total or partial knee replacement (see chapter 16).

RHEUMATOID ARTHRITIS

While osteoarthritis attacks the knee's articular cartilage, rheumatoid arthritis (RA) begins in the synovial tissue. This autoimmune disorder strikes earlier in life, usually in both knees, and affects more women than men. While there is no cure for RA, there are many ways of treating it to relieve symptoms and diminish the extent of permanent damage to your knees.

Diagnosis

In addition to a comprehensive physical examination, a blood test can determine if you have rheumatoid factor (RF), an antibody made by your immune system. This is often present in someone with RA. X-rays of your joints will help rule out other forms of arthritis. X-rays are taken over the years to track the progression of the disease. MRI can be very useful in determining the extent of rheumatoid synovitis and assessing your response to treatment.

Treatment

Medication, weight control, and exercise are the primary forms of treatment for rheumatoid arthritis. Rheumatologists prescribe a number of pain medications for RA, including NSAIDs, COX-2 inhibitors, corticosteroids, disease modifying antirheumatic drugs (DMARDs), immunosuppressants, and biologic response modifiers, as well as antidepressants. (See chapter 14 about medications.)

In advanced or recalcitrant cases of RA, a synovectomy may be necessary to "debulk" the extensive synovial tissue in the joint. Using arthroscopic techniques, the surgeon removes the inflamed joint lining. This can help to manage symptoms, but it is not a permanent cure. In cases of aggressive RA with extensive joint damage, knee replacement may be required to help maintain mobility and function.

JUVENILE RHEUMATOID ARTHRITIS (JRA)

Juvenile rheumatoid arthritis is less common than the adult version, but it is very similar in symptoms and treatment.

Diagnosis

JRA is essentially diagnosed and treated the same way as adult RA but under the direction of a pediatric rheumatologist.

Treatment

NSAIDs, one type of medication used to reduce pain and inflammation, should never be given to children without a doctor's direction. Regular exercise and physical therapy are generally prescribed to help a child maintain flexible and strong muscles to protect the knees and other joints. Nutrition is also important to maintain a child's overall health with a balanced diet that includes calcium to promote bone health. The pediatric rheumatologist is an expert in the treatment of this condition and will utilize different classes of medications to assist patients in maintaining joint health and function for as long as possible.

SEPTIC ARTHRITIS

Septic arthritis (see chapter 4) is caused by a bacterial infection. When it strikes the knee joint, it causes the same symptoms as other forms of arthritis, but it also causes systemic symptoms such as fever, chills, and an elevated white blood cell count.

Diagnosis

In addition to a comprehensive physical examination, your doctor may perform the following blood tests to check for systemic signs of infection: complete blood count (CBC), C-reactive protein (CRP), and erythrocyte sedimentation rate (ESR). If joint infection is suspected, your doctor will aspirate fluid from your knee to send to the lab to determine the extent and type of infection. The white blood cell count and differential (the types of white cells present) are extremely useful in diagnosing acute septic arthritis. A bone scan or MRI is often performed to see if the infection has spread to the adjacent bone.

Treatment

Septic arthritis is treated with surgical drainage of the knee joint and intravenous antibiotics. The infected synovial fluid is removed from your knee through arthrocentesis, a simple procedure that involves inserting a needle into your knee joint to drain the fluid and relieve the pressure on your knee. This is followed by arthroscopic surgery to remove the thickened synovial tissue and to wash out the infected parts of your knee. Antibiotic therapy is initiated as soon as a specimen has been taken for a bacterial culture. Patients are usually started on a combination of antibiotics until the exact type of bacteria and its sensitivity to particular antibiotics is determined.

Following surgery, gentle exercises will begin to help keep your knee from getting stiff. Most acute knee infections can be eradicated, but stiffness is common after such infections.

PSORIATIC ARTHRITIS

As explained in chapter 5, you won't get psoriatic arthritis unless you have psoriasis. This disease is more common in adults than children. Most people have the skin symptoms before they are diagnosed with the arthritis.

Diagnosis

The same diagnostic tools—X-rays and blood tests—are used to diagnose psoriatic arthritis as have been described for other types of arthritis.

Treatment

Psoriatic arthritis cannot be cured, but treatment can control inflammation, and prevent pain and further damage to the knees. Treatment varies based on the pattern of joint involvement. There are several types of medications that may be used to treat psoriatic arthritis, including NSAIDs, corticosteroids, disease modifying antirheumatic drugs (DMARDs), immunosuppressant drugs, and biologic response modifiers known as TNF-alpha inhibitors.

In addition to topical medications, continued treatment of the skin condition involves preventing dry skin by avoiding strong soaps or chemicals, using nondeodorant soaps, putting baby oil in bathwater, and using a humidifier in winter.

GOUT

Needlelike crystals of uric acid that are deposited in the joint spaces of the knees (and big toe) cause gout (see chapter 5), an inflammatory type of arthritis.

Diagnosis

In addition to a comprehensive physical examination, a blood test is needed to identify the presence of hyperuricemia. Because elevated uric acid may not always be present in gout, it is necessary to aspirate (drain) the knee fluid to look for the presence of uric acid crystals and make a definitive diagnosis of gout. These crystals have a very characteristic appearance under a microscope.

Treatment

The goal of treating gout is to stop the acute flare, eliminate the risk factors for future acute attacks, and manage the chronic pain associated with the disease. The first line of treatment is to restrict foods that provoke attacks of gout (see page 64) and to reduce alcohol consumption. Allopurinol may also be prescribed to block uric acid production. This drug comes in tablet form and is taken once a day. Colchicine is another medication used as a maintenance therapy for gout. There are medical contraindications to these medications, and it is important to discuss the pros and cons of their use with your doctor.

Prevention

One way to prevent gout is to keep uric acid levels down.

- Do not drink alcohol, because it interferes with the removal of uric acid from your body.
- Drink plenty of water to help your kidneys excrete uric acid.

- Maintain a healthy weight to avoid stress on your knees, but avoid any rapid weight loss program (especially high protein diets) that can increase your uric acid levels.
- Avoid foods high in purines.

PSEUDOGOUT

Pseudogout is also called chondrocalcinosis or calcium pyrophosphate deposition disease (CPPD). It is caused by an excess of calcium pyrophosphate crystals that are deposited in the knee joint, rather than uric acid as in regular gout. Although it is unclear why, the crystals deposit in the synovium, meniscus, and articular cartilage (chondrocalcinosis). It is not known whether the deposition of these crystals causes joint degeneration or whether the crystals deposit in areas of existing degeneration.

Diagnosis

Pseudogout is not the same as gout but is sometimes confused with that disease because it can produce similar symptoms of pain, swelling, and inflammation during an acute flare. However, calcium pyrophosphate deposition can also be seen in older patients who have minimal symptoms. In addition to a comprehensive physical examination, your knee fluid may be aspirated and tested for the presence of calcium pyrophosphate crystals, which have a characteristic appearance under the microscope. Moderate deposits of these crystals can be seen on X-ray.

Treatment

There is no treatment to dissolve the calcium pyrophosphate crystals. NSAIDs may help pain and swelling, but if for any reason you cannot tolerate them because of poor kidney function or gastrointestinal problems, intermittent corticosteroid injections can help manage acute flares. The condition often improves on its own, although some people have recurring attacks. If you have two or more attacks a year, your doctor may recommend a low dose of colchicine.

TEN WAYS TO KEEP YOUR ARTHRITIC KNEES AS PAIN FREE AS POSSIBLE

Lifestyle changes may help slow or even prevent knee pain from inflammatory conditions. There are steps you can take to avoid or limit the extent of disability. Overall advice is to maintain your ideal weight, stay active in a smart way, and build muscles that support your knees.

1. Maintain a healthy weight so that you place less strain on your knees and delay cartilage breakdown. The best way to control weight is by increasing nutrients while limiting calories. This can be done by eating more fruits and vegetables and less saturated fat and simple carbohydrates. If your weight is a problem, ask your doctor to recommend a program or consult a nutritionist. Rapid weight loss often results in rapid weight gain. It is often necessary to change your food and eating lifestyle slowly to achieve success.

2. Keep moving. Recent studies show that physical activity does not make arthritis worse. In fact, if you are sedentary, you are twice as likely to lose mobility in everyday life as people who are active. Physical activity helps the supporting muscles, increases blood flow to the knee, and stimulates and nourishes the underlying cartilage. However, avoid or limit participation in activities and sports that cause pain. Low-impact activities like walking, cycling, water aerobics, swimming, and tai chi are good options.

3. Exercise regularly. Exercise alone can help relieve many of the symptoms of arthritis, including pain and fatigue. Low-impact exercise performed on a regular basis can help distribute the synovial fluid, a kind of natural motor oil that helps keep the joint moving smoothly. Hip and gluteal buttocks muscles get weak from sitting, which can leave the knee more vulnerable. Exercise your hip abductors and gluteal muscles. Stretch and strengthen the quads and hamstrings. Use weights to strengthen muscles around your knees. (See chapter 18 on conditioning.)

4. Use cold packs. Cold has a numbing effect that can help manage arthritis pain. Apply cold several times a day for fifteen to twenty minutes. Some people prefer to briefly massage the painful area with an ice cube. If you do this, keep the ice moving to avoid frostbite. (See chapter 12 on conservative treatment.)

5. Use heat. Heat will relax tense muscles and can help relieve pain. Try an electric heating pad on the

low setting. Be sure to place a towel between your skin and the pad. Do not fall asleep with a heating pad on, as you can burn yourself. You can also use a heat lamp, or inexpensive gel-filled pack, or try soaking in a warm bath.

6. Get a massage. New studies show that traditional Swedish massage can help alleviate the pain of arthritis of the knees by making the knees more limber and encouraging walking. (See chapter 17 for more about massage.)

7. Use proper body mechanics. Changing the way you perform everyday tasks can make a tremendous difference in how you feel. Proper posture when sitting, lifting, standing, turning, and walking can help protect your knees. (See chapter 19.)

8. Pace yourself. Battling pain and inflammation can leave you feeling exhausted. Divide exercise and work activities into short segments and rest before you get tired. Find time to relax during the day. An appropriate level of activity should make you feel the same or better afterward, not worse. Introduce new activities gradually and heed warning signs. If you experience pain later in the day or fatigue the following day, you've done too much.

9. Learn to manage stress. The chemicals that your body releases when you are under stress can help you deal with demanding situations. But the downside is that they can suppress your immune system and may worsen the inflammatory condition. Trying to cope with worsening symptoms may make you feel even more stressed,

setting up a destructive cycle. While you can't eliminate all stress from your life, you can learn to manage it. Exercise, deep breathing, and comforting rituals like afternoon tea are some examples of techniques to lower stress.

10. Maintain a strong support system. Friends and family can help you face the physical and psychological challenges of arthritis pain. Just having someone to talk to may help, and support groups composed of other people with the same condition may be beneficial. Call the local chapter of the Arthritis Foundation (see appendix) to find a support group. You can also ask your doctor, because many medical centers have affiliated support groups.

KEY POINTS

- Treatment of osteoarthritis depends on age and general health, but includes rest, icing, physical therapy, and medications, along with lifestyle changes such as weight loss, regular exercise, and avoiding activities that cause pain.
- The most popular oral supplement for treating symptoms of osteoarthritis is a combination of glucosamine and chondroitin sulfate.
- Only in advanced cases is rheumatoid arthritis treated with synovectomy, a surgical procedure to remove the inflamed joint lining.
- Juvenile rheumatoid arthritis (JRA) is generally treated with medication and regular exercise.

- Septic arthritis must be treated with antibiotics, as well as the same pain management used for other forms of arthritis.
- Gout is treated by avoiding risk factors such as alcohol and foods high in purines, as well as with pain management.
- Many lifestyle changes can reduce the pain of arthritis, such as exercise, weight loss, proper nutrition, and stress reduction.

Chapter 11

Treating Chronic Knee Pain from Other Medical Conditions

There are several diseases that cause knee pain, and the underlying disease must be treated. For example, Lyme disease, which is caused by a tick bite, can result in painful knees years later. Benign tumors can form in the lining of the knee and cause considerable pain and discomfort. Primary bone cancer, while less common than other cancers, does affect the leg bones and knees more often than other parts of the body. Children are more vulnerable than adults to these cancers, and they are also at risk for Blount's disease, which can cause the legs to bow.

LYME DISEASE

Manuela was a nineteen-year-old seasonal farm worker from Ecuador who spent summers at the farms of New England. When harvest was over, Manuela returned home to her family. There she came down with what she thought was a virus. The doctor in her hometown questioned her but didn't associate her condition with anything she may have encountered while in New England. Nevertheless, he gave her some antibiotics, which helped her overcome her "virus." However, Manuela developed arthritis in her knees two years later. While working in the field in Connecticut, she began having trouble with swelling and stiffness. She was afraid to give up her job, so she went to a doctor, who, after taking a history and physical exam, asked if she had ever noticed a tick bite.

Most people would not associate a tick bite—especially if they did not know they had it—with painful knees years later. Untreated Lyme disease can cause inflammation and joint pain, particularly in the knee, and can lead to arthritis. Late stages of the disease may develop months or even years later, making it more difficult to diagnose.

About half the people with late stage Lyme disease develop episodes of swelling and pain, sometimes with redness, in a few large joints, especially the knee. About 10 percent of people with Lyme disease arthritis develop persistent knee problems. Numbness and shooting pains in the back, legs, and arms may also occur. A smaller number of people develop neurologic abnormalities, including problems with mood, speech, memory, and sleep.

Lyme disease is caused by the spirochete *Borrelia burgdorferi*, which is usually transmitted to people by deer ticks. Children and young adults who live in wooded areas are most often infected by ticks in the summer and early fall. It was not until 1975, when a cluster of cases occurred in Lyme, Connecticut, that the disease was identified. Today it is the most common insect-borne infection in the United

States, occurring in forty-seven states as well as in Europe and Asia. However, 80 percent of cases occur along the northeastern coast, from Massachusetts to Maryland.

After a tick bite, spirochetes multiply at the site of the bite, and after a few days they migrate into the surrounding skin and spread through the blood to other organs and joints, such as the knees. Once the disease spreads throughout your body, you may feel ill with flulike symptoms such as fatigue, chills and fever, headaches, stiff neck, and aches in muscles and joints. Less common symptoms include backache, nausea and vomiting, sore throat, swollen lymph nodes, and an enlarged spleen. Most symptoms come and go, but feelings of illness and fatigue can last for weeks. Symptoms are often mistaken for influenza or common viral infections, especially if there is no history or usual evidence of a tick bite. Some people get more serious symptoms, such as abnormalities of nerve function, facial weakness, an irregular heartbeat, or chest pain.

Diagnosis

Knee pain from Lyme disease is difficult to diagnose unless your doctor thinks about the possibility. Many people who live in areas where Lyme disease is common have painful knees, but for other reasons. Diagnosis is especially problematic if you don't recall a tick bite, or your doctor doesn't connect the two conditions. It is often a diagnosis of exclusion, when no other source of pain is found, and blood tests for Lyme disease are performed. If you live in an area with deer and spend time outdoors gardening, hiking, or exercising, you should alert your physician.

Proper diagnosis depends on both test results and the

presence of typical symptoms in a person who lives in or has visited an area where the disease is common. Most commonly used tests measure antibodies to the spirochete in the blood. However, these alone are not enough because they are often negative in early stages of the disease, and sometimes positive in those who do not have it.

Treatment

Lyme disease is treated with oral or intravenous antibiotics, and early treatment is the best way to prevent complications. Some people will have persistent arthritis even after Lyme disease is treated and cured, and may need NSAIDs to control pain.

PIGMENTED VILLONODULAR SYNOVITIS (PVNS)

Pigmented villonodular synovitis (PVNS) is a benign tumor in the synovium of the knee. It may show up with swelling or knee pain, with repetitive episodes of locking, or you may notice a mass in your knee.

Diagnosis

PVNS is often misdiagnosed initially. In addition to a physical examination and history, your doctor will want to investigate any unexplained, recurrent fluid in the knee, especially if the fluid is rust colored, which raises the suspicion of PVNS. This diagnosis is confirmed with MRI, which is very useful in defining whether the PVNS is the nodular or diffuse type. Nodular PVNS is an isolated mass of PVNS tissue that is well localized. This type often causes locking, a loose-body symptom. The synovial fluid is generally normal in appearance. In diffuse PVNS, all or part of the lining of the knee joint is involved. This type will generally appear with unexplained swelling, and the synovial fluid may be rust colored. When PVNS causes no symptoms, your doctor may discover it when you have an MRI or arthroscopy for an unrelated problem.

Treatment

The treatment for PVNS is surgical, and it varies depending on your overall health, age, medical history, and the extent and location of the tumor. Because PVNS may continue to grow and invade the surrounding tissues, the synovial tissue must be surgically removed in a procedure called synovectomy (see chapter 15). Before arthroscopic techniques, open surgery was used to perform a complete synovectomy. It is sometimes still necessary to perform open surgery for cases of diffuse PVNS that have invaded tissues outside of the capsule of the knee.

Arthroscopy has vastly improved this surgery. When PVNS afflicts the cruciate ligaments that crisscross in the front and back of your knee, the synovial membrane must be dissected away from the ligaments. Because it requires such skill, it is always important to find the best orthopedic surgeon you can. The chance of recurrence is based on both the successful removal of the tissue and characteristics of your case that may result in a more or less aggressive tumor.

The nodular form of PVNS is less likely to recur, while the diffuse form has a high risk of recurrence. PVNS is not considered malignant, but it recurs in half the cases, so your doctor may recommend a follow-up MRI to monitor for recurrence. In some severe cases, treatment with radiotherapy is indicated. If PVNS is uncontrolled for years, it may result in significant destruction of the joint, and knee replacement may be necessary.

BLOUNT'S DISEASE

Blount's disease in children needs to be diagnosed and treated early to prevent it from getting progressively worse and leading to permanent disability. (See chapter 11.)

Diagnosis

A physical exam will determine that a child's lower legs are bowed. If the child stands with feet touching together and has a significant gap between the inner sides of the knees, Blount's disease is considered. An X-ray of the knee and lower leg confirms Blount's disease. If only one leg is involved, a comparison view of the other knee will be obtained.

Treatment

If Blount's disease is detected before a child is three years old, it can usually be corrected with bracing. If bracing fails, or if the disease is not detected until a child is older, surgery may be needed to reestablish symmetrical growth of the tibia. When surgery is indicated, the growth of the outer side of the tibia can be surgically restricted to allow the child's natural growth to reverse the bowing process. This procedure is called an epiphyseodesis, and it promotes premature fusion of the lateral part of the physis. A staple or small plate is applied across the lateral growth plate to stop that growth and allow the medial growth to "catch up." This less drastic surgery is most effective when there isn't too much bowing, and the child still has a significant amount of growing to do. Once surgery has restored the legs to normal appearance and function, and both are properly aligned, the child can return to normal activities and sports. In some children, the disease may recur after surgery.

Failure to treat Blount's disease may lead to progressive deformity. If Blount's is present on only one side, this will result in a discrepancy in leg length and an abnormal gait.

BONE CANCER

Primary bone cancer is treated by an oncologist and orthopedic surgeon with training in surgical oncology.

Diagnosis

Bone and knee pain and swelling can be from any number of conditions, most of which are not cancer. Your past medical history and physical exam, in addition to X-ray, bone scan, CT scan, and MRI, will help your doctor formulate a diagnosis.

If a secondary bone tumor is suspected, your doctor may want to order a bone scan to see if any additional sites are tumor present. A bone scan consists of the injection of a radioactive tracer into your bloodstream, which will collect in areas of abnormal bone. Your doctor can then use a special camera to determine abnormal sites. A bone scan can help to localize the area of a tumor and determine if the tumor has spread to other sites in the bone.

A CT scan is often carried out to evaluate the spread of the tumor outside of the bone. Once your doctor has a good idea of the location, spread, and possible type of tumor, a biopsy is performed to obtain a specimen of tissue that can be analyzed to diagnose the type of tumor. Your doctor will perform the biopsy using a needle to remove a small piece of tissue from the tumor, or with a surgical incision to remove a portion of the tumor itself (see chapter 7 about diagnostic tests).

Treatment

The specific treatment for bone tumors depends on a number of factors, including age, overall health, medical history, type of tumor, the extent of local spread, and whether or not the cancer has metastasized. Treatment can include surgery, chemotherapy, radiation, and amputation.

Surgery is the most common treatment for primary bone cancer. The aim is to remove the tumor along with a margin of healthy tissue around it. In the past, amputation of the limb was common, but advances in surgery, chemotherapy, and radiation have decreased the need for this. Treatment may also include supportive care (for the side effects of treatment), prosthesis design and fitting (in the case of amputation), and long-term follow-up with a physician to monitor response to treatment, to detect tumor recurrence, and to manage any long-term complications related to the initial treatment.

The treatment of bone cancer is beyond the scope of this

chapter. If this diagnosis is made, it is very important that you find the right treatment team of oncologist and orthopedic surgeon to help you with this condition. Your medical team will educate you and your family concerning the diagnosis, the medical and surgical treatment options, and your short-term and long-term prognoses.

KEY POINTS

- Knee pain caused by arthritis that developed from undetected Lyme disease is treated with antibiotics.
- A surgery called arthroscopic synovectomy is generally required to treat pigmented villonodular synovitis (PVNS).
- If Blount's disease is detected early, it can be treated with bracing.
- The surgical procedure for Blount's disease will restrict growth of the outer side of the tibia to reverse the bowing. This is called epiphyseodesis.
- Treatment for bone cancer includes a variety of techniques, such as surgery, chemotherapy, and radiation.

PART III

TYPES OF TREATMENT FOR KNEE PAIN

Chapter 12

Conservative Treatment

Jake is a do-it-yourself guy. He prides himself on making all the repairs on his house and his car, and most times he does a pretty good job. So when he hurt his knee by falling down hard after getting twisted up in a hose he had left tangled on the patio, he figured he would fix it himself and get back to work. He sat down in his lounge chair, put on the TV to catch the rest of the ball game, and put a heating pad on his knee. But Jake's pain got worse, his knee got red and swollen, and to make matters worse, his team lost. What did Jake do wrong? Well, he forgot that heat stimulates blood flow and relaxes muscles, while ice soothes pain and inflammation. And at the time, forcing more blood into his painful knee was the wrong thing to do.

RICE: FIRST AID FOR KNEES

For all knee injuries, your first treatment should be RICE, a well-known acronym for rest, ice, compression, and elevation. These four steps also help relieve pain from chronic conditions such as arthritis, tendinitis, muscle sprains, and bursitis, and symptoms following surgery or trauma.

Over-the-counter NSAIDs, including aspirin, ibuprofen, and naproxen do help to relieve pain and inflammation. Not everyone can safely use NSAIDs, though, so it is important to discuss this with your doctor and to follow the package recommendations. If you are not able to use NSAIDs, acetaminophen (Tylenol) can help pain but has no effect on inflammation.

Rest

Rest your knee. If it's difficult to walk, or you are limping, stop putting any pressure on your knee. It won't heal or feel any better if you keep using it, so take a break from regular activities. For a minor injury, you may need only a day or two of rest, but more severe damage—such as a sprained ligament—will take longer and will likely require medical attention.

Ice

Ice will reduce both the inflammation and the pain in your knee and should be applied every hour for twenty minutes following an injury. When chronic pain caused by inflammation becomes intense, you may want to apply ice—but less frequently. Whether you use a store-bought cold pack, ice from your freezer, or a bag of frozen vegetables to cover your knee, place a dry towel between your skin and the ice to protect your skin from ice burn. Ice therapy is effective, but don't leave ice on your skin too long at one time because you could damage the nerves in your skin or the skin itself. If the area becomes numb to the touch, you should remove the ice because you have lost protective sensation. It is possible to develop frostbite from overly aggressive use of ice. After a couple of days of ice therapy, you may want to switch to heat to relax your muscles and increase blood flow to your knee.

Compression

Compression can help decrease swelling in your knee by preventing fluid from building up in the damaged tissues (edema). Use a lightweight and breathable elastic, such as an Ace bandage, to wrap your knee. It needs to be tight enough to support your knee but should not be so tight that it causes your calf or foot to swell below the wrap.

Elevation

Elevate your knee to allow gravity to drain away any fluids that may accumulate after an injury. This will help alleviate swelling. If you have a recliner, that would be a comfortable and effective way to elevate your leg. In order for elevation to be helpful, the injured area must be at least at the level of your heart. Prop your leg up when in bed by putting pillows under your ankle and lower leg. Don't put a pillow only under your knee, as it might make it more difficult to straighten your knee after a period of prolonged knee flexion.

PROTECTION: BRACE YOURSELF

Some doctors like to add a *P* for protection and turn this into PRICE. Protection with a brace, for example, may sometimes be necessary to protect your knee from further injury. There are many kinds of knee braces made from a wide assortment of materials. They come in a variety of sizes, colors, and designs. The purpose of a knee brace is to support the structures of your knee while you are recovering from an injury. It can also be used to provide support to diminish the risk of injuries and, in some cases, reduce pain. There are four main kinds of knee braces:

- Prophylactic braces to protect your knee from injury during sports such as football.
- Functional braces that support your knee if it has already been injured.
- Unloader braces that augment treatment for osteoarthritis.
- Patellofemoral braces that improve patellar tracking and relieve anterior knee pain.

You may need more than one type of brace, depending on what the problem is. For example, you may need a rehabilitative brace after ACL reconstruction surgery to support your knee, and later a prophylactic brace to protect it from reinjury. Knee braces are only aids; they do not offer you 100 percent protection from future injury.

You also need to learn how to wear a brace properly, so always ask your doctor or physical therapist to demonstrate how to put it on and use it correctly. Straps, tapes, hinges, and hooks all have to be properly fastened, or the brace may not do its job. Exposed metal needs to be covered to protect others who may come in contact with your knee if you are using the brace during team sports. Knee braces can usually be cleaned with soap and water.

Prophylactic Knee Braces

Prophylactic knee braces were originally designed to protect the knee ligaments from contact or sports injury. The design of these braces includes an elastic neoprene sleeve with hinged bars on either side of the knee. For optimal protection, the hinge needs to be correctly placed at the level of your knee joint. Prophylactic braces were tested by the National Football League to prevent injury, but their initial popularity has diminished as effectiveness (and cost) is questioned. At best, such braces help resist lateral knee impact but don't provide protection against rotational stress that harms the cruciate ligament.

A brace may offer a sense of protection during contact sports, but it is less important than strength training, conditioning, and flexibility in protecting knee ligaments.

Functional Knee Braces

A functional knee brace is designed to provide stability to your knee after an ACL, PCL, or other ligament injury, and it may decrease your risk of sustaining another. These braces, too, were initially marketed to athletes as a means to prevent injury, but they are more widely used by people who have had reconstructive surgery—to reduce strain on the grafted ligament—or by people who have opted not to undergo ligament reconstruction. Functional knee braces come in standard sizes but can also be custom made for better fit. Your doctor will give you a prescription for such a brace after ligament injury or reconstruction. The brace also needs to be fitted by a trained orthotist, because a poorly fitted brace may not be helpful. Discuss the use of functional braces with your doctor and physical therapist. There is tremendous variability in the use of braces following ligament surgery, and the decision is highly individual. Your sport, your knee anatomy, and the status of your ligament will all be factors that drive the decision to use or not use a functional brace.

While there is still no definitive scientific evidence, many people who use functional knee braces say the brace has helped stabilize their knee and made them feel more confident, while others find such braces to be too confining.

Unloader Knee Braces

Osteoarthritis is often more prevalent in the medial (inner) compartment of the knee joint. The unloader brace shifts weight bearing from the inside toward the outside of your knee and, thus, reduces pain. The brace works by changing your gait. Several studies of unloader knee brace use show that many people have significantly less pain and improved physical function when wearing it. The unloader can also improve posture and enable people with osteoarthritis to walk longer distances. In some cases, using this brace along with medical treatment can prevent or delay the need for knee replacement surgery. While this brace can be used to unload either the medial or lateral compartments, use in medial compartment arthritis is most common.

Patellofemoral Braces

Pain in the front of the knee is common in active people of all ages, but it can also be a symptom of a misaligned patellofemoral joint. Patellofemoral braces range from easy-to-use, inexpensive braces, like an elastic sleeve with a cutout hole for your patella, to more complex braces designed to alter patellar tracking.

These braces can help your muscles support and control the position of your patella and can reduce pain. There is some scientific data that patellofemoral braces can ease the pain of patellar subluxation, but users' responses vary, so discuss this first with your doctor. The simple braces are available in sporting goods stores and pharmacies, while complex braces require a prescription and careful fitting.

KEY POINTS

- Rest, ice, compression, and elevation (RICE) help relieve acute knee pain and swelling.
- Always see a doctor if first aid does not resolve your knee pain or swelling within twenty-four to forty-eight hours.
- If you are unable to bear weight on your injured knee, or if you heard a pop or snap at the time of injury, seek medical attention immediately.
- Several types of knee braces are available to protect and support your knee after an injury or surgery.
- It is important to discuss the use of bracing with your doctor following a significant knee injury or surgery.

Chapter 13

Physical Therapy

Remember Anna in chapter 2, the short, overweight woman who fell down and broke her knee in three places? She had open surgery to repair her kneecap and then faced months of physical therapy to rehabilitate her knee. This included strengthening the muscles around her knee—as well as her back, leg, and ankle muscles. The fall and subsequent surgery and use of a walker and cane made Anna feel like an invalid, and she was determined to overcome this. And she did. She was religious about her therapy, and her knee improved dramatically, much sooner than expected. The surgeon was surprised at the speed with which Anna rehabilitated herself. She also went on a weight management program and took off the sixty pounds that had been adding pressure to her knee.

Sam, fifty-six, was also in physical therapy, but he was there before his surgery. By strengthening his quads and hamstrings before having ligament reconstruction, he was ensuring a quicker recovery.

Physical therapy is guided exercise that is frequently part of your medical treatment for arthritis, trauma, or other painful knee conditions. It is also a critical part of the rehabilitation process following knee injury and surgery. Physical therapists focus on educating you about your knees, relieving pain and swelling, restoring range of motion and flexibility, and strengthening the muscles in your thighs, calves, and hips, and core abdominal muscles. A course of physical therapy can help:

- strengthen your muscles to support your knee;
- improve your flexibility, mobility, and balance;
- teach you better ways to use your body in everyday life;
- improve fitness to reduce the risk of recurring injury;
- improve chronic knee pain;
- prepare your body for surgery so that your recovery is quicker;
- help your body recover from injury or surgery;
- recondition you after major knee surgery;
- prepare you to return to sports or an active lifestyle.

Your doctor will prescribe physical therapy as part of your medical treatment and will work with a licensed physical therapist to design a phased treatment plan. Some of these exercises may require special equipment and machines. Therapists may also use hot and cold packs, ultrasound, deep tissue massage, and electrical stimulation. Your therapist will also train you in the use of assistive devices such as canes, crutches, and braces.

Your physical therapist will know your medical history. Before beginning a program, he or she will perform a comprehensive evaluation to assess your range of motion, strength, balance and coordination, posture, and motor function. In the early stages of rehabilitation, physical therapy reestablishes your knee's full range of motion. You will then progress to exercises to strengthen knee, hip, and ankle muscles. This is combined with training to improve your stability and balance. Finally, you will work on training specific to your occupation, lifestyle, or athletic activity, including exercises to help you prevent further injury.

Depending on your knee condition, age, and gender, it can take a variable amount of time to return to your normal activities. For example, if you had a simple arthroscopy for a meniscus tear, you might go to physical therapy for four to six weeks. In contrast, recovery from an ACL reconstruction or knee replacement could take six months to a year.

Most importantly, keep in mind there is no "one size fits all" protocol for each particular knee condition. Just because your friend with arthritic knees is advised to walk on a treadmill at a certain speed and incline does not mean that is what you should do. Physical therapy is very personal, and your program fits only you.

MEETING YOUR PHYSICAL THERAPIST

Most orthopedic treatment centers have a physical therapy department on-site or have working relationships with therapists in your community.

A physical therapist must be licensed by the state—every

state in the nation requires this—before he or she can practice in a hospital, clinic, or private office. These therapists can treat you at home, in your hospital room, or in a clinic. Education requirements are increasing. Where a master's degree was considered enough in the past, the trend now is moving toward therapists' earning doctoral degrees in physical therapy. In addition to basic science and health, physical therapists receive training in specialized courses in the anatomy of the nervous system, examination techniques, therapeutic procedures, and human growth and development. They now receive additional training in radiology and other medical areas that can affect what they do. Physical therapists may also select a specialty such as geriatrics, pediatrics, or sports medicine, and receive additional training and certification in those areas.

Physical therapists consider themselves "rehab specialists," and they are in charge of how your day-to-day rehabilitation is done. Your therapist will see you over and over again, spending much more time with you than your doctor. Thus, your therapist may have a better sense of how your condition is improving and what still needs to be done. For example, your doctor may estimate that you should be off your crutches in six weeks, but your therapist, who looks at your whole body while you walk, is able to gauge whether or not you are ready to give up the crutches.

Look for a therapist who maintains a close relationship with your doctor, one who will consult with the doctor about your orthopedic evaluation, surgery, and other medical treatment. For example, your therapist needs to know about the quality of your bones, or just how widespread is the arthritis in your knee, or what type of graft was used for your ligament reconstruction. Always ask your physical therapist about whether he or she is communicating regularly with your doctor and providing the doctor with progress reports.

Never confuse the role of a personal trainer with that of a physical therapist. Personal trainers generally do not have medical training. They are educated to varying degrees in physical fitness, but this is not the same as physical therapy.

YOUR ROLE IN YOUR PHYSICAL THERAPY

Physical therapy is your part-time job as a patient, and you need to be active in your own rehabilitation. You are getting better not only because of your physical therapist but because you are following your therapist's guidelines and changing the way you use your body outside of your therapy sessions. Whether you go to physical therapy daily or only once a week, your therapist will give you exercises to do at home between sessions. Do your homework! This helps keep your blood flowing and your muscles flexible, so that the work you do in your therapy session is not lost during your time away. Think of your therapist as a highly educated medical coach to lead you through a course of action to achieve your goals for comfort and lifestyle.

Your therapist will also educate you about modifying certain activities as you recover from your injury or surgery. It is important to follow your therapist's suggestions. If you are working out in addition to therapy, let your therapist know about your level of activity, and once your prescribed physical therapy is complete, ask your therapist to suggest a program of exercise that you can follow for the rest of your life.

AIDS TO PHYSICAL THERAPY

A good physical therapist can treat you in an empty room without the aid of any special equipment. He or she will be able to assess what you need by watching you perform any number of activities, such as walking, bending, or stepping on a stool. However, a physical therapy center may have many fitness machines and various types of equipment that can augment the basic therapy of how you are using your body. Basic physical therapy is aided by some of the following:

Fitness Machines and Equipment

Any number of machines and fitness equipment may supplement your basic physical therapy, but they are not the primary component of treatment.

Hydrotherapy: Walking and exercising in a swimming pool puts less strain on painful knees, and this is something that you can continue on your own if you have access to a swimming pool. A person with crutches can usually walk more easily underwater, so an underwater treadmill may be used at the physical therapy center.

Stationary bicycles: Arthritic knees are often helped on bikes with a short crank, which means your knee does not have to bend as far as a normal bicycle crank.

Elliptical trainer: This combination treadmill and stair climber is an excellent fitness machine for painful knees.

Treadmill: Speed and incline can be adjusted to suit individual needs. Sometimes walking backward on the treadmill is used to train the quadriceps for deceleration exercises such as walking downstairs.

Balance equipment: There are a variety of implements that can help you develop better balance and coordination. These include balancing on a big foam pillow or learning to stand—and eventually balance—on a disk that wobbles. (Never try these without supervision from your physical therapist.)

Therapeutic Massage

Therapeutic massage is often a routine part of a prescribed physical therapy program, especially for treatment of a soft tissue injury. It can help to decrease muscle spasms, improve muscle flexibility, and guide and restore range of motion after trauma, overuse injury, or an operation. Following knee replacement surgery, for example, massage can help to break up any scarring of the knee tissue that may limit motion. Sometimes this massage may be painful, so it is usually followed by treatment with ice to reduce pain and swelling. (See chapter 17 for more about massage.)

TRANSCUTANEOUS ELECTRICAL NERVE STIMULATION (TENS)

Physical therapists sometimes use transcutaneous electrical nerve stimulation, or TENS, as part of a rehabilitation program and as a way to reduce knee pain. It is an adjunct to treatment to reduce pain or swelling, or to build up the quadriceps. It is not the key component. You need the basics first, such as modifying activity that causes pain.

TENS uses electrical impulses applied to the skin

through small EKG-like electrodes to diminish the processing of pain impulses. TENS also increases the release of
endorphins, brain chemicals that act as a sort of natural
painkiller. While it is not a cure for pain, it may relieve
symptoms in some people. It is often used by physical therapists to provide several hours of pain relief for those suffering from rheumatoid and osteoarthritis, and for some
postsurgery pain. However, TENS is best used in conjunction with other therapies, such as medication. You cannot
use TENS if you have a pacemaker or during pregnancy.

PAYING FOR PHYSICAL THERAPY

Most health insurance plans, including HMOs, are required
to cover physical therapy treatment. However, there is
significant variability in what types of medical conditions
qualify for physical therapy coverage, how much of the cost
will be covered, and for how long. Sometimes coverage
applies only for a certain number of treatments during a
calendar year. You need to know ahead of time what the de-
ductible may be and how much of the cost you will have to
pay yourself.

Many states have recently passed direct-access legislation
that permits you to see a physical therapist without a prescription from a physician for a limited time or number of
sessions. Not all insurance companies will reimburse for
direct access care, so it is important to check your policy.

Also, check your insurance coverage to see if physical
therapy is covered for more than one condition. For example, you may be getting physical therapy for a spinal disor-

der in addition to what you will need for your knee surgery. It is also important to understand whether or not the therapy is covered until normal function is restored to your knee. If you are covered for only a limited number of sessions or time period, it may not be enough to restore function following an ACL reconstruction. Some insurance covers thirty visits per calendar year or thirty visits per diagnosis, so it is critical that you know what your plan includes. While payment to your orthopedist may be covered, you need to be sure that the recommended physical therapist is also covered by your insurance.

Physical therapists not only manage your treatment, but how you pay for that treatment. The therapist sends your evaluation and recommended treatment to the insurance company and they will work together on how best to use the allotted visits. You and your physician and therapist need to know how to work this out.

KEY POINTS

- Physical therapy is the use of exercise and physical treatment methods to relieve pain and restore function to your knees.
- Make sure that the physical therapy program designed by your orthopedist or physiatrist is performed in conjunction with a physical therapist licensed in your state.
- Massage, electrical stimulation, manual resistance, fitness machines, free weights, and strength training equipment are often a part of physical therapy treatment.

- Do your physical therapy homework exercises consistently to keep the momentum of your treatment going.
- Check with your insurance company to see how many physical therapy visits you are allotted and work with your therapist to design the best possible program to fit within that allotment.

Chapter 14

Treating Knee Pain with Medication: Balancing Benefits with Side Effects

Peter never liked taking pills, or any kind of medicine, for that matter, but his knee pain was bothering him more, so he consented to take a prescription NSAID that his doctor recommended. He was told to take a pill every six hours and to time it so that the last one was just before he went to bed. But Peter was typical of many people. He did not take the pills as directed, but took them only when his pain was severe. Had he taken them as directed, he might have felt little or no pain at all. Peter did not understand that dosages are timed for a reason. Because Peter waited until his knees hurt, he had to wait another forty-five minutes to an hour for the pill to kick in.

Medication can help relieve pain, but it is important to understand how medications for knee pain work and what you can expect from different types. Prescription medication is useful only if your doctor prescribes it appropriately and you take it according to the directions. There are also numerous over-the-counter medications and nutritional supplements used to treat knee pain or injury.

Oral medications used for knee pain include what we refer to as NSAIDs (nonsteroidal anti-inflammatory drugs), COX-2 inhibitors (a special subtype of NSAIDs), acetaminophen, rheumatic medications, and narcotic pain medications. Over-the-counter medications such as aspirin, ibuprofen (Advil, Nuprin, Motrin), and naproxen (Aleve) fall into the class of NSAIDs but are available at lower dosages than their prescription counterparts.

Injectable medications such as corticosteroids and viscosupplements such as Synvisc and Hyalgan are also used to treat knee pain.

Many people with knee pain use glucosamine and chondroitin, MSM (methylsulfonylmethane) fish oil supplements, and nutritional preparations. Many of them may be safe. But it is very important to understand that while these remedies are available without prescription, they are not regulated by the U.S. Food and Drug Administration (FDA).

Your goal should be to find the least invasive way of getting the best pain relief with the least side effects—and all drugs have side effects. Very often, through careful trial and error, and by trying several different medications, you can achieve excellent pain control with few or minor side effects.

TIMING AND METHOD OF DELIVERY

Timing the dosage correctly is as important as finding the correct medication. If you know a pill takes forty-five minutes to work, don't wait until your knee pain is severe to take it. Anticipate what you are going to do and take your pill before you take a walk, play with the kids, or go shopping, so that the medicine will be in effect before you begin to stress your knee. This may also help keep your dosage down.

Drug delivery, the process through which a drug enters your body and begins to work, can take time. When you take a drug by mouth, it takes approximately forty-five minutes to be digested and absorbed. Some of the medication may be broken down by the digestive process or passage through the liver, so less of it is available to diminish pain. Injecting medication under the skin (subcutaneously) or into the bloodstream (intravenously) is more efficient than pills but also more invasive. Drugs introduced directly into the bloodstream deliver the medication more quickly to reduce pain impulses within the central nervous system. In fact, drugs administered by the subcutaneous or intravenous route are three to six times more potent than the same dose given by mouth.

Aspiration and Injection

An injection of medication directly into your knee allows still less drug to be given with fewer side effects. Aspiration and injection can be done with the same puncture to alleviate knee pain.

Aspiration removes fluid from your knee and allows your doctor to look at the fluid and send it for analysis, if needed. An acutely injured knee will be filled with blood. If your doctor sees fatty material in the blood, it indicates that a fracture or other damage to the bone within the knee has occurred. Clear, thick yellow fluid is generally seen in people with osteoarthritis, cartilage or meniscus injury. Cloudy fluid can be seen with gout, pseudogout, inflammatory arthritis, and infection. In this case, your physician will send the fluid to a lab to look for evidence of crystals, inflammation, or infection.

Injection of medication into the knee can be a rapid and safe way to get relief because it allows the doctor to put the drug directly at the site of the disease and avoid some of the potential toxicities of that medication if it were taken orally. The needle inserted into your joint is similar to those used to draw blood from a vein. Your physician will carefully clean the area where the needle is inserted, to decrease the risk of infection. A cold spray such as ethyl chloride may be applied to your skin to temporarily decrease the sensation of the puncture. You will feel some momentary pain when the needle is injected, but it is minimal if you are relaxed.

The two most common medications injected into the knee are corticosteroids and viscosupplementation fluids. The benefits of a corticosteroid shot can last for months in an arthritic knee; it can be useful in managing inflammatory knee conditions.

NONSTEROIDAL ANTI-INFLAMMATORY DRUGS (NSAIDS)

NSAIDs may reduce pain and inflammation in your knee. At the right dosage, these drugs may be effective in treating the pain of arthritis, inflammatory conditions, trauma, and overuse injury. Many NSAIDs are sold over the counter in low dosages that do not require a prescription. The most common NSAID is aspirin, but ibuprofen and naproxen are also available without a prescription.

It is important not to confuse aspirin with Tylenol, which is acetaminophen, *not* an NSAID. Though Tylenol can control pain just as well as NSAIDs—without their risk of gastrointestinal problems such as stomach upset, heartburn, and ulcers—acetaminophen doesn't have any anti-inflammatory properties. For many people with painful knees, Tylenol can be used to control pain as a first-line drug combined with applications of ice. For conditions with both pain and inflammation, the judicious and short-term use of NSAIDs can be very helpful.

Side Effects

NSAIDs have potential side effects that can occur with short-term or long-term use. You should never take more than your doctor recommends. In some people, even small doses can cause stomach pain, nausea, ulcers, and stomach bleeding. There is also what is called a "ceiling effect" with NSAIDs. This means there is a limit to how much pain they can actually control. For example, if you have moderate to severe knee pain, it won't help you to take more of the drug than is recommended—and it won't help to combine several different types of NSAIDs. In fact, it is *dangerous* to take NSAIDs in combination, so never take more than one at the same time. The one exception to this can be the use of baby aspirin (used for cardiac symptoms) and NSAIDs. This must be discussed with your doctor before combining these medications, to insure your safety.

At high doses or with prolonged use, particularly in women over sixty-five, NSAIDs can cause nausea, indigestion, and ulcers. They can also bring about liver and kidney damage, elevate blood pressure, and lead to mild water retention. This water retention can be enough to put some people with frail hearts into heart failure. At any dose, all NSAIDs interfere with the ability of the blood to clot. That's why you must stop taking them ten days before surgery or invasive procedures to restore your normal blood-clotting mechanism.

Drug companies have come under more intense scrutiny from the Food and Drug Administration in recent years, and they now must provide more information on labels about possible cardiovascular or gastrointestinal side effects. Always read the label before taking any medication, whether it is by prescription or over the counter. Discuss any potential concerns with your doctor. It is important to check with your doctor to see if the new medication has any impact on other medications you are currently taking.

How to Use NSAIDs Effectively

If one type of NSAID does not work, you may want to try another. Some people respond well to ibuprofen, while others see a better response with naproxen or aspirin. Always read the label on the box to determine the safe and most effective dose. If you take an NSAID for two weeks without benefit, then you need to see your doctor. If you are using over-the-counter NSAIDs on a regular basis, please discuss this with your doctor. It may be necessary to monitor your blood levels to check for side effects. Ask your doctor about taking higher doses of the over-the-counter medication or using a prescription NSAID.

Also available by prescription are COX-2 inhibitors, which are a more selective NSAID. These medications, such as Vioxx, Bextra, and Celebrex were thought to have fewer gastrointestinal side effects but may have other side effects. Vioxx and Bextra were taken off the market because of reported increases in cardiac events in the people using them. Celebrex and Mobic are still available, but they must be prescribed by a physician who has a good understanding of your medical history. The FDA has asked the manufacturer to review its drug label to include warnings about the possible cardiovascular and gastrointestinal side effects. It's best to use COX-2 inhibitors and NSAIDs for the shortest possible period and at the lowest possible dose.

NUTRITIONAL SUPPLEMENTS

The breakdown of joints in arthritis results in production of certain bodily substances—prostaglandins, among others—that irritate the synovial membranes that line the joint. These structures contain a rich supply of pain receptors. Many people with arthritis pain seek alternative solutions because NSAIDs and Tylenol just don't do the job.

Glucosamine and chondroitin are substances found naturally in cartilage and are available without prescription as nutritional supplements. Unlike NSAIDs, which reduce inflammation, glucosamine may act to relieve pain and may slow down the rate of cartilage destruction. However, there is no scientific evidence that these supplements can make articular cartilage regenerate.

Glucosamine is a nutritional supplement that can help reduce *mild* pain in many patients with arthritis and other musculoskeletal pain. This supplement is derived from the shells of crab, lobster, and shrimp. It is marketed as a treatment to enhance growth of cartilage and has no known toxicity, but there is no clear scientific evidence of its benefit in the long run. It has not proven helpful for people with severe arthritis.

Chondroitin, another nutritional supplement, is a component of normal cartilage and is often used in combination with glucosamine. Studies on chondroitin are fewer than those for glucosamine, and any added benefit of chondroitin to glucosamine remains to be determined.

Glucosamine *may* help knee pain caused by wear and tear or even osteoarthritis when taken in combination with chondroitin. When participants in a study who had moderate to severe knee pain from arthritis took chondroitin plus glucosamine, they had more relief—and no additional side effects—compared with a placebo (a sugar pill), or the COX-2 inhibitor Celebrex.

It is reasonable for people suffering from arthritis pain to try a six-to-eight-week course of a supplement such as CosaminDS, which contains both supplements. If you are uncertain whether it is helping, stop taking it after two months and monitor your symptoms. If you haven't gotten relief after eight weeks, save your money and stop the supplement. And if you do feel better, taking a break from the supplement will reveal whether your pain has gone into remission, which can happen with arthritis. If pain recurs, you can restart the supplements.

Keep in mind that nutritional supplements are not regulated by the FDA; therefore, consumers have no way of assessing the product's purity or knowing how much of the active ingredient(s) it contains. Read labels carefully and discuss your use of supplements with your physician.

TOPICAL PAIN RELIEVERS

People have long applied skin ointments, such as Bengay, to relieve sore muscles. Some medical researchers are studying this effect on painful knees. A 2004 study published in the *Journal of Rheumatology* reported that Celadrin, a cream made with cetylated fatty acids, helped relieve knee pain from osteoarthritis within thirty minutes. Another study using a lidocaine patch on arthritic knees also showed significant relief.

In other countries, topical NSAIDs are recommended by physicians for chronic conditions such as tendinitis and arthritis. They are thought to be as effective as oral NSAIDs but without the side effects. Topical diclofenac gel has been studied by German medical scientists on people with osteoarthritis of the knee. Pain is relieved by applying a gel to the knee four times a day. This is an alternative medication that may provide relief to those who cannot tolerate oral pain relievers. Topical formulations of many nonsteroidal anti-inflammatory medications are found in Europe, but none of these drug formulations is approved by our Food and Drug Administration for use in the United States to date.

There are over-the-counter products sold here that may help provide temporary relief of knee pain. Arnica is a salve made from an herb grown in the mountain regions and is sometimes known as Arnica montana. There are several brand names available. Another topical remedy, one made with capsaicin, may provide temporary relief of arthritis pain. This salve, made from an ingredient in chili peppers, is sold under many names, and some pharmacies make their own brand.

VISCOSUPPLEMENTATION

Viscosupplementation entails injecting a painful arthritic knee joint with an artificial fluid that mimics natural synovial fluid. Hyaluronic acid (HA) is a component of the thick fluid found in healthy joints. This material is made from rooster combs and was originally used to treat racehorses. In 1997 the FDA approved injectable HA for use in treatment of human arthritis, although medical scientists still are not quite sure how it works. This material can be injected into arthritic knees and may ease pain. The HA is made by a number of companies and is injected into the knee once a week as part of a series of injections. Some forms of the substance require three injections; others up to five. This medication does not have the side effects of oral medications, so it may be appropriate if you are unable to take other medications or if they are not helping your arthritis pain. HA injections have been reported to provide pain relief for six months to a year, but the treatment does not (to our knowledge) slow down progression of arthritis. Though this therapy is well tolerated, there have not been any long-term studies yet. Some patients have a very positive response, while others do not see much improvement. Some people experience a local inflammatory reaction at the injection site that will cause pain and swelling. If this occurs after an injection, be certain to call your physician.

CORTICOSTEROIDS

Corticosteroids are man-made drugs that are chemically similar to cortisol, a hormone produced by the adrenal glands. Because they reduce inflammation and swelling, they can be used to treat joint pain. They are far more powerful than NSAIDs, but so are their potential side effects. Corticosteroids to treat osteoarthritis are most commonly administered by way of a local injection. This allows a low dose of medication to be used and decreases potential side effects. A selective injection of corticosteroid into an arthritic or inflamed joint can be extremely useful in managing pain. The injectable form still has side effects, including elevated blood sugar levels in diabetics and an increased risk of infection. Corticosteroids can be taken orally, but this route is generally used for people with systemic arthritis affecting multiple joints. Because oral use of corticosteroids can affect the entire body, the risks are more significant.

Side effects from oral corticosteroids by mouth initially include insomnia, mood swings, ulcers or esophageal reflux symptoms, increased appetite, and menstrual irregularities. Diabetics will see their glucose levels rise, and some people who are not diabetic may become so while taking steroids.

If you take corticosteroids for more than a few weeks, you may gain weight, develop acne, and retain fluid with swelling of the legs. As time passes, the side effects also include increased risk of infections due to diminished immunity. A change in the distribution of fat can occur with chronic steroid use, resulting in a hump over the back of the lower neck. Other side effects include osteoporosis, muscle weakness (particularly in the thighs), and breakdown of the skin.

Obviously, all these side effects compromise the body, so use these medications only when absolutely needed and for as short a duration as possible. These are potent medications and must be prescribed carefully by your physician. If oral corticosteroids are prescribed for you, it is important to discuss their pros and cons with your doctor. Many rheumatic causes of knee pain will require prolonged use of corticosteroid therapy. The use of oral corticosteroids in treating other knee conditions is extremely rare.

DISEASE MODIFYING ANTIRHEUMATIC DRUGS (DMARDS) AND BIOLOGIC RESPONSE MODIFIERS (BIOLOGICS)

If you have rheumatoid or psoriatic arthritis, your rheumatologist may prescribe disease modifying antirheumatic drugs (DMARDs) or biologic response modifiers (biologics) to treat the underlying autoimmune disease that causes your knee problems.

DMARDs slow down or prevent the immune system from attacking the knees, which in turn prevents swelling and pain. These drugs can be very effective in stopping the progression of joint damage, but they can't repair existing damage. The most commonly prescribed DMARDs include leflunomide, methotrexate, sulfasalazine, and hydroxychloroquine.

Biologics are a new class of genetically engineered drugs that block immune system molecular pathways that cause inflammation. They are often used in combination with DMARDs like methotrexate and are typically administered intravenously in a clinic or given as injections at home. Because these drugs suppress the immune system, they must be used very cautiously in anyone who is prone to infections. Biologics include adalumimab, etanercept, and infliximab. They are also called TNF blockers. TNF (tumor necrosis factor) is a cytokine, or cell protein, that acts as an inflammatory agent in rheumatoid arthritis, and these drugs block that agent.

Both DMARDs and biologics have tremendous potential to change the course of inflammatory arthritis. The development of these medications has shifted the treatment away from the use of chronic high-dose corticosteroids to a treatment protocol that will halt progression of the disease. These medications are prescribed by rheumatologists with considerable expertise in their use, side effects, and anticipated clinical outcomes.

SAFE USE OF NARCOTIC PAIN MEDICATIONS

Narcotic pain medications are usually reserved for the severe pain that follows surgery. If you remain in the hospital after surgery, you may be given pain medications that you can control yourself as you need it. This is called patient controlled analgesia—PCA—a method of reducing postoperative pain. If you have outpatient surgery, you may be given prescription pain medications such as Percocet, which are effective in alleviating pain but cannot be used long term.

Knee pain rarely needs to be treated with narcotics. Exceptions to this are acute fractures, severe ligament injuries, and postsurgical pain. Fear of addiction should not prevent you from getting pain relief with effective and timely use of these drugs. In a 1999 survey conducted for the American Academy of Pain Medicine and the American Pain Society, 49 percent of those who had taken narcotic pain relievers said they were concerned about addiction. Yet the data show that the vast majority of patients with pain do not become addicted to narcotics when used appropriately for acute pain. Most orthopedic conditions require only short-term use of narcotic pain medications. Use of chronic or high-dose medication should be done only in consultation with a pain management specialist.

Here's how your body reacts to narcotics:

Tolerance means that your body adapts to a narcotic so that it has fewer therapeutic benefits and side effects. Fortunately, tolerance to the side effects develops relatively quickly, but tolerance to the pain-relieving effects of these drugs develops more slowly. Most chronic pain may be treated with a stable dose of medication, once the pain is controlled.

Dependence is your body's adaptation to the continued or repeated presence of a narcotic. In the absence of the drug for a period of time, your body will go into withdrawal. The withdrawal symptoms from narcotics can be severe, and sudden cessation of the chronic pain medication should be done under medical supervision. Dependence and tolerance are normal physiological adaptations to the exposure of the central nervous system—and the body—to a chemical on a regular basis.

Addiction is using a drug for the purpose of seeking

pleasure—to get "high." Addiction to and abuse of prescribed narcotics occur in about the same percentage of people that engage in other substance abuse. In general, narcotics are effective medications for the treatment of severe acute pain and are safe pain relievers when taken appropriately. If you have concerns about using any medication, be sure to talk with your doctor.

KEY POINTS

- It may take some trial and error with medications to find the one or combination that brings the greatest relief with the least side effects.
- NSAIDs have potential gastrointestinal side effects.
- Common medications for treatment of knee pain include oral medications such as NSAIDs, COX-2 inhibitors, and acetaminophen.
- Timing pain medication correctly can help you control your knee pain.
- Injectable treatments such as corticosteroids and viscosupplementation can help you manage arthritis pain in your knees.
- Taking narcotics as prescribed for short periods to control pain does not commonly lead to addiction.
- Let your doctor know if you are using over-the-counter medications, including nutritional supplements, in addition to your prescribed medications.
- Never share prescription medications and never give your prescription medications to a friend.

Chapter 15

Treating Knee Pain with Arthroscopic and Open Surgery

Many people think that once their knees become painful or arthritic, they will just get new knees. They may be unaware that there are many types of surgical procedures that can be done to knees to avoid or delay such a drastic event. For example, you can have "plugs" of cartilage implanted in your knee to treat localized cartilage loss. Or, if osteoarthritis is on one side of the knee, an osteotomy can realign the knee to switch the pressure to the other side and relieve the pain.

Knee surgery is necessary to repair or reconstruct torn ligaments and tendons, to repair or remove menisci, to remove abnormal synovium, loose fragments of bone or cartilage, and to correct abnormal alignment or instability of the kneecap. Many surgical procedures today are performed with arthroscopic techniques and often on an outpatient basis. Open surgery, generally requiring a stay in the hospital, is needed for some procedures, such as complex multi-ligament reconstructions and knee replacement. Other procedures, such as patella realignment and cartilage restoration, require a combination of arthroscopy and small open surgical incisions.

Since the late 1970s, when modern arthroscopic knee surgery was first developed, better arthroscopic lenses and higher-resolution cameras have improved the accuracy and effectiveness of the procedure. Knee arthroscopy is now one of the most common orthopedic procedures in the world. Using a fiber-optic light source, a thin lens, and a camera, surgeons can create a high-resolution image on a television monitor to evaluate the joint and to perform surgical procedures through tiny incisions.

Arthroscopic knee surgery can be done under local anesthesia (just the knee), regional anesthesia (lower half of the body), or general anesthesia (unconscious). Two or three very small incisions called portals are made in the knee. A tube is placed through one portal in order to pump a sterile saline solution into the joint. This fluid expands the space—like blowing up a balloon—to make room for the camera and small manual or power-driven instruments such as scissors, clamps, shavers, and lasers. Your surgeon will thoroughly inspect all of the structures inside the knee joint, including the articular cartilage, menisci, and ligaments. The normal and abnormal areas are usually photographed to provide a record of the status of your knee and what was done. Several different surgical procedures can be performed via the same three incisions, from flushing out loose bits of damaged cartilage to reconstructing ligaments. When surgery is completed, the incisions are closed with sutures or paper tape and covered with a bandage.

Depending on the complexity of the procedure, arthroscopic surgery can take from fifteen minutes to several hours. Arthroscopy is the term for the surgical technique that is used to perform many different procedures inside the knee. Often people will compare themselves to a friend who had arthroscopic knee surgery, but it is important to understand that many different injuries and conditions, some more or less complicated, can be treated with this procedure.

Most people recover quickly from arthroscopic surgery and can go home the same day, but some procedures require a hospital stay to manage postoperative pain. Whether your surgery is outpatient or inpatient depends on your condition, the type of surgery, your general health, and your doctor's preference. While arthroscopy is less invasive than open surgery, it is still surgery. Depending on your injury and what was done to your knee, you may need pain medication, crutches, a brace, special care at home, and rehabilitation with physical therapy. Be sure to discuss with your surgeon what you can expect after the surgery.

WHAT TO ASK YOUR DOCTOR BEFORE KNEE SURGERY

Assuming that you have already done your research and chosen the surgeon you feel is best for you, there are still many questions to ask. You need to know how your lifestyle will be affected following surgery, whether or not you will be able to drive, if and how long you may need crutches, or how much assistance you will need at home.

When you discuss potential surgery with your orthopedist, be sure to ask these questions:

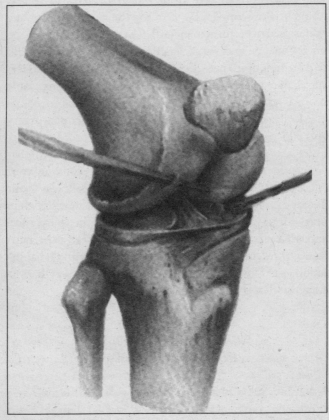

FIGURE 4. Orthopedic surgeons make tiny incisions in the knee in order to insert a fiber-optic light and camera as well as the instruments needed to perform a variety of surgical procedures, from reconstructing ligaments to flushing out loose bits of cartilage. (© *Olga Spiegel, 2007.*)

- How will this surgery help my knee condition?
- May I see an illustration or skeletal model of what is wrong with my knee and how it will be fixed?
- Do I really need this surgery, or might I get by with a less invasive treatment?
- What will happen if I choose to delay surgery?
- What are the pros and cons of surgery?
- What are the side effects and possible complications of this surgery?
- What is the recovery like, and how long before I am back to normal?
- How should I prepare for lifestyle changes after surgery?
- Will I be able to walk?
- Will I be able to drive a car?
- Will I be able to climb stairs?
- When may I anticipate returning to work?
- How many of these procedures have you performed?

GETTING READY FOR SURGERY

Whether you have arthroscopy or open surgery, including knee replacement, there are things that you can do to prepare yourself. If you are over age forty or have any chronic conditions, such as hypertension, you may need a complete physical examination prior to surgery to ensure that your health is good enough to go through with the operation.

The extent of the preoperative evaluation is based on your medical history, age, and complexity of the surgical procedure. The preoperative medical evaluation and testing can range from something as simple as a blood test to a much more thorough evaluation including a chest X-ray, EKG, and medical assessment. If you are having a total knee replacement, you may also be asked to donate your own blood prior to surgery in case a transfusion is needed during or after the procedure.

If you take medications for other medical conditions, your surgeon or primary care physician will let you know which to continue until surgery and which need to be discontinued. For example, you will be asked to stop taking aspirin and other NSAIDs five to seven days before surgery because they can increase the risk of bleeding. It is very important to tell your doctors about any herbal or other supplements that you are taking. You might not think of these supplements as drugs, but they can affect your health and your response to other medications.

Another important consideration before knee replacement surgery is the condition of your teeth. Dental disease is often a source of bacteria entering the bloodstream. Before you have a knee replacement, you will need to treat any significant dental problems, including tooth extractions or periodontal disease.

Be certain that your doctor is aware of allergies or sensitivities to any medications, latex, or tape. Before going to the hospital, discuss postsurgical care with your doctor and family. Meet with your physical therapist to plan ahead for your postoperative visits and be sure to get your pain medication prescription in advance so that you can begin immediately after surgery.

In most circumstances, you won't be able to eat or drink anything after midnight the night before surgery. If your operation is scheduled for late in the day, this restrictior may change. Be sure to discuss this with your surgeon. If you eat or drink when you should not, your surgery may be postponed or canceled. You will be told by the hospital or facility when to arrive at the hospital. This is frequently two hours before your scheduled surgery. Bring loose shorts or sweatpants that will fit comfortably over your knee bandage when you leave.

Anesthesia

There are many different techniques used to provide anesthesia for knee surgery. The type of anesthesia depends on your knee condition, your age and medical health, and the facility where your surgery is performed. At the time that you discuss surgery with your orthopedist, you can get a sense of what is customary for your surgery. More detail will be provided by a member of the anesthesia team, who will discuss the use of local, regional, or general anesthesia. The anesthesiologist will make a recommendation concerning the best approach for your surgery and will discuss risks and side effects of the different types. If you have local or regional anesthesia and are having an arthroscopic procedure, you may be able to watch the procedure on the TV monitor.

- Local anesthesia is an injection of anesthetic into the knee and portals that numbs the immediate area. It is often combined with intravenous sedation to relax you.
- Regional anesthesia means that a region of your body will be anesthetized for the surgery, such as epidural anesthesia, the most common. With this,

you can't feel anything below the waist, but you can
be awake or sedated, depending on your preference.
- General anesthesia keeps you unconscious during
  the surgery and will require the use of a ventilator
  to assist in your breathing.

     Throughout these procedures, the anesthesiologist
will monitor your blood pressure, respiration, and
oxygen levels, regardless of whether you are having
local, regional, or general anesthesia.

MENISCUS SURGERY

The meniscus is the disc-shaped pad between your femur
and tibia. A meniscectomy is the surgical removal of a torn
section of meniscus. If a meniscus tear is causing pain, locking, or swelling, the torn pieces need to be removed and the
edges shaved smooth. Whether the surgeon decides to remove or repair a meniscus tear depends on the location,
length, and pattern of the tear; the overall condition of
the meniscus; and your age. For example, tears at the outer
edge—the red-red zone—where there is a good blood supply, can often be repaired. The inner two-thirds of the
meniscus have less potential to heal with surgery because of
the variability of the blood supply.

     The meniscus plays an important role in the knee, so
your surgeon will attempt to save as much of it as possible.
The ability of your surgeon to repair your meniscus is also
affected by the complexity of the tear. Be sure to ask your
surgeon about any lifestyle limitations you may have after
meniscal repair surgery.

The amount of time it takes you to recover from meniscus surgery depends on your knee characteristics and the type of tear. For example, a partial meniscectomy in an otherwise healthy knee is a straightforward procedure with an estimated recovery time of approximately six weeks. You may need to keep weight off your knee with crutches or a cane and take NSAIDs for the first few days to minimize postoperative swelling and pain. Physical therapy is often recommended following surgery. Some people may be on crutches for up to six weeks and may also need a brace to limit range of motion following meniscal repair. Full recovery from meniscus repair can take three to four months. If you have lost a significant amount of meniscus and have persistent pain, your surgeon may recommend a meniscal transplant using a donation from a tissue bank. This is a complex procedure with a long recovery, and is not the right choice for everyone.

ARTICULAR CARTILAGE SURGERY

Articular cartilage cannot regenerate and usually thins out with age. Osteoarthritis is a direct result of worn-out articular cartilage. In younger people, articular cartilage is most frequently damaged from injury. Medical treatment and exercise can help ease pain, but over time, many people will undergo knee replacement surgery. However, in people too young to consider replacement, there are other surgical treatments to consider.

Cartilage Debridement

Cartilage debridement is an arthroscopic surgical procedure that removes the fragments or flaps of damaged articular cartilage from your knee when it has been damaged from injury. Removing damaged tissue may prevent the injury from extending into the healthy tissue. Leaving a large cartilage flap or area of damaged cartilage in the knee can result in mechanical symptoms such as catching or locking. However, cartilage debridement is a palliative treatment. That is, it helps reduce pain, but it does not cure or restore the underlying area of cartilage loss.

Microfracture

Microfracture restores the gliding articular surface of your knee joint by creating tiny openings in the bone at the base of a cartilage defect. First the calcified cartilage layer adjacent to the bone is removed. Then, with an awl, tiny fractures are created in underlying bone, and bleeding occurs from these holes. Multiple perforations are made into the bone at the site of the cartilage loss in order to make it bleed. There are stem cells in the blood and bone that seep out of the openings. The body reacts to these microfractures as if they were injuries, and this is why new fibrocartilage grows. It has characteristics of both cartilage and scar tissue.

This procedure of microfracture has been used for more than twenty years to encourage the spontaneous repair of tissue. It is a relatively quick procedure—it takes about thirty to forty-five minutes—and is minimally invasive, with a success rate of about 75 percent to 80 percent among people ages forty-five or younger. The recovery time is based on the size and location of the treated area.

To optimize formation of the fibrocartilage following the procedure, a CPM (continuous passive motion) machine is prescribed for use six to eight hours a day for the first six weeks. This keeps your leg moving without any effort on your part. Depending on the location of the treated area, you may need crutches or a brace during this time. With the help of physical therapy, most athletes can return to sports in about six months.

Microfracture is used to treat localized cartilage injuries and has become a popular procedure in the sports world in recent years. It is less effective in treating older people, those who are overweight, and those with severe cartilage damage. It is not recommended for anyone with osteoarthritis or large areas of cartilage loss.

Mosaicplasty

Mosaicplasty, also known as osteochondral grafting, is used to treat people with cartilage damaged from trauma or arthritis. It is a type of cut-and-paste procedure designed to replace lost cartilage and bone on the surface of the knee joint by implanting osteochondral plugs (plugs of cartilage and bone). The plugs can be your own (autograft) or from a tissue bank (allograft) and are grafted into damaged areas of articular cartilage. Cores of cartilage and bone measuring three to eight millimeters are removed from areas of the knee that are exposed to less daily load and are transplanted into the site of cartilage loss. There is a limit to the number of plugs that can be taken from the knee. If the area of cartilage and bone loss is too large, allograft tissue can be used.

According to scientific studies, mosaicplasty may be a long-lasting as well as cost-effective way to treat local cartilage defects.

Autologous Chondrocyte Implantation (ACI)

Autologous chondrocyte implantation is a cell-based cartilage replacement therapy. The only FDA-approved procedure of ACI in the United States is Carticel, which is used only for the treatment of young, healthy people with limited damage to their articular cartilage. The treatment is not designed for treating osteoarthritis.

This is a two-stage surgical procedure. In the first stage, biopsies of healthy articular cartilage containing thousands of your own cartilage cells (chondrocytes) are removed from your knee using arthroscopic techniques. This material is sent to Genzyme laboratories, where the cells are isolated, grown in culture, and multiply for six weeks. Then, in a second, open surgical procedure, the multiplied cells—now in the millions—are put back into your knee and held in place with a small patch of tissue. The implanted cells then divide and integrate with the surrounding tissue to create more cartilage.

ACI is an extremely expensive procedure ($20,000 to $35,000), and only about 1,500 to 3,000 are performed each year in the United States. The results of ACI are similar to microfracture, but early results show that this procedure may be more durable. More research is underway to simplify the procedure and to minimize the trauma associated with the need for open surgery.

SYNOVIUM SURGERY

A synovectomy is a surgical procedure that removes the inflamed or diseased lining (synovium) of your knee. This can help relieve pain in the early stages of rheumatoid arthritis, and it is also used to remove benign synovial tumors such as PVNS (see chapter 5).

The diseased synovium is removed either with small shavers connected to suction or by cauterizing the tissue—using heat to destroy it. Arthroscopy has vastly improved this surgery, but, nevertheless, it remains a lengthy and exacting procedure requiring a highly skilled and experienced surgeon.

A synovectomy is not curative, as it is impossible to remove every synovial cell. In many cases, the synovium will grow back. The goal of synovectomy is to remove as much of the abnormal synovium as possible, which may allow improved medical management. Your knee may be swollen for many weeks, so always follow the recommendations of your physician and physical therapist to keep discomfort to a minimum. Physical therapy after synovectomy is essential to regain strength and range of motion.

LIGAMENT RECONSTRUCTION SURGERY

Reconstruction of the ACL is the most common arthroscopic ligament reconstruction because a complete tear of the ACL rarely heals. Surgery replaces the torn ligament with a soft tissue graft from your own body (autograft) or from a tissue bank (allograft).

The type of graft used is highly individual, based on your

age, gender, history of prior knee injury, your sport, and your activity level (see chapter 5 about ligament injuries). The recommended graft type also depends on your surgeon's expertise.

Scientific studies indicate that there is no clear difference in outcome between hamstring and patellar tendon autografts. The data comparing autograft and allograft continue to be compiled. There have been changes in allograft harvest and graft sterilization techniques over the last five to ten years but long-term data are not yet available.

- Autograft surgery requires a small open incision to harvest a piece of your patellar or hamstring tendons. The graft is pulled through tunnels created in your tibia and femur and is placed in the same position as your natural ACL. The graft is held in place with screws or other fixation devices made of metal, plastic, or synthetic materials that are slowly absorbed by the body. These devices are required to hold the graft in place until it heals strongly to the surrounding bone. New blood vessels will grow into the transferred graft and help it heal. In addition to your arthroscopy portals, one or two small incisions are made to harvest your graft and to create the bone tunnels.
- Allograft has become increasingly common because it eliminates the pain caused by harvesting a graft from your own body. Allografts can come from several tendons: patellar, hamstring, Achilles, or tibialis anterior (front of the tibia). Allografts are taken from cadavers and processed with the best current scientific techniques, but there is the

potential for transmission of infectious diseases.
In addition, the long-term outcome of allografts is
unknown.

Ask your doctor about the latest information before you
decide on a choice of graft.

ACL reconstruction is not an emergency surgery, so you
have time to get yourself prepared mentally and physically.
It is usually performed on an outpatient basis and has vastly
improved over the last decade, with a better understanding
of pre- and postoperative rehabilitation. The goal of this
procedure is to restore knee stability, which is important in
decreasing your risk of subsequent cartilage and meniscus
injury once you return to an active lifestyle.

Most orthopedists will prescribe exercises for you to do
before surgery. These are extremely important in order for
you to regain your full range of motion and strength before and after surgery. Although it is less common now than
ten years ago, some physicians will prescribe a continuous
passive motion (CPM) machine to help with range of motion in the first week following surgery. This moves your
knee very slowly to decrease the risk of stiffness and loss of
motion. Ask about this before surgery, because your doctor
may have a preference.

Rehabilitation

After reconstructive surgery, you will need to wear a long
leg brace and walk on crutches for a week to ten days to diminish swelling and to protect your ligament reconstruction as it heals. There is a lot of variability among surgeons
about how much weight bearing is permitted after surgery.

Applications of ice and elevating your leg as often as possible will help control swelling. NSAIDs and narcotic pain medication will help manage your postoperative pain.

Home exercises will begin shortly after surgery so that you can learn how to take care of your knee and strengthen your leg while protecting the new ligament (see chapter 13 on physical therapy). In order to prevent your knee from getting stiff, your physical therapist will teach you how to bend and straighten it (out of the brace) several times a day. As the swelling decreases, and your knee gets stronger, you will be able to walk without crutches and work on getting your whole leg strong and your knee stable.

Supervised physical therapy can begin two to fourteen days after surgery and continue for three to six months, depending on your age and activity level, your surgeon, and the type of graft. Once supervised physical therapy is completed, you can move on to a program at your local gym or health club. The majority of active people who have an ACL reconstruction return to sports or activities that require rapid pivoting or changing direction by six months. Some athletes may have a more accelerated rehabilitation, and others may progress more slowly.

There is tremendous variability in the postoperative rehabilitation protocols that doctors prescribe. These protocols generally evolve over time, based on a surgeon's experience, graft choice, and patient population. There are no large scientific studies showing that one rehab protocol is superior to another, so review your plan thoroughly with your surgeon. If you are struggling with your recovery and physical therapy, ask your therapist to talk with your surgeon.

The reconstruction of the PCL is done with a similar

procedure using autograft or allograft. Reconstruction of the LCL and MCL must be performed with open surgery, as those ligaments are on the outside of the joint and cannot be visualized or reconstructed using arthroscopic techniques.

REPAIRING RUPTURED PATELLA AND QUADRICEPS TENDONS

The patellar tendon connects your patella to your tibia. It can be ruptured by a sports injury in people under forty, but most commonly occurs with a slip or fall on a bent knee. Such ruptures can also be a complication of knee replacement or of ACL reconstruction when part of the tendon is removed to use as a graft. Some ruptures result from chronic patellar tendinosis (jumper's knee); others may be the final result of chronic tendon degeneration from a history of injury; and others occur after corticosteroid injections.

Rupture of the quadriceps tendon, which attaches the quadriceps muscle to the upper edge of the patella, also typically occurs with a fall. This injury is sometimes missed initially if small portions of the quad tendon remain intact, and it is more common in people over age forty.

With appropriate diagnosis and treatment, surgical intervention may restore normal knee function. Repair of a patellar tendon or quad tendon rupture is performed with open surgery, as these structures are technically outside the knee joint. A series of strong sutures are woven through the tendon and passed through small tunnels in the patella. This allows the tendon to be reattached to the bone.

Patella and quadriceps tendon repairs must be protected for the first six weeks following surgery with the use of a long leg brace or splint. Physical therapy can progressively restore knee range of motion, patella mobility, and strength. Full recovery can take six to nine months, but knee stiffness is a common complication of tendon repair surgery.

OSTEOTOMY

An osteotomy may be an alternative to total knee replacement in younger people with arthritis in either the inner (medial) or outer (lateral) compartment of the knee joint. If you have osteoarthritis on only one side of your knee, this surgical procedure can shift the weight load to the healthier side. Shifting the alignment of the bones can slow cartilage degeneration, relieve pain, and improve function and, for some, helps delay the need for knee replacement. This procedure is usually performed in younger and more active people to relieve pain and restore knee mobility. An X-ray of your legs performed while you are standing will reveal whether or not you are a good candidate for an osteotomy. This X-ray will include your hip, femur, knee, tibia, and ankle, and is designed to measure the alignment of your knee joint.

There are two techniques for performing a tibial osteotomy: opening wedge or closing wedge. Both require a four-to-five-inch incision over the upper third of the tibia. Your surgeon will map out the wedge of bone to be removed, or opened, then use an oscillating saw to create a controlled, well defined "fracture" across the tibia.

- A closing wedge high tibial osteotomy removes a small wedge of bone from the lateral tibia, shifting the load-bearing axis of your knee from the damaged medial side to the healthy side so that arthritic surfaces are no longer taking all the load. An appropriately sliced bone wedge is removed, and the wedge is closed, changing the shape of the tibia and the alignment of your knee joint. This shifts the knee from a varus (bowleg) to a valgus (knock-kneed) alignment. The osteotomy site is then stabilized with a plate and screws.

- An opening wedge high tibial osteotomy will change the bony alignment by opening up a triangle of bone. This technique helps to maintain the length of your tibia but requires use of a bone graft or bone graft substitute to fill the opening created. The "fracture" is created, and the bone is wedged open to create the desired angle. Then a plate and screws are attached to stabilize the osteotomy. Because this technique creates a gap in the bone, bone grafting is needed.

- A femoral osteotomy can also change the alignment of your knee, but this technique is performed much less frequently than high tibial osteotomies. It is used for excessively knock-kneed people with lateral (outer) compartment arthritis. A controlled fracture is made in the end of the femur above the knee joint. The change in alignment is made, and a plate and screws are used to stabilize the osteotomy.

After all osteotomy surgeries, the soft tissues are closed, and a bulky compression dressing is applied. These procedures can take one to two hours and are often performed in combination with arthroscopic debridement. You will likely remain in the hospital for a day or two for pain control following surgery.

Your leg will look different after surgery as it heals into its new alignment. Your weight bearing status and need for a brace will depend on the type of procedure, the stability of the osteotomy, your bone health, weight, and your surgeon's preference. Osteotomy relies on bone healing before more vigorous weight bearing exercise can be done. Therefore, you will need X-rays at regular intervals while the osteotomy site heals, so your surgeon can monitor your progress. Osteotomy surgery will slow but not stop the progression of knee arthritis. Conversion to a total knee replacement may be needed ten to fifteen years after corrective osteotomy.

PATELLOFEMORAL SURGERY

Patellofemoral surgery treats a variety of conditions such as patellar tilt, subluxation or dislocation, and isolated patellofemoral arthritis. All are meant to correct the angle or function of the kneecap. These surgical procedures are performed arthroscopically or with open surgery, depending on the underlying problem and the extent of the surgery needed.

Lateral Release

A lateral release is an arthroscopic surgical procedure that corrects patellar tilt. In some people, the bands of the lateral retinaculum, a supporting ligament that controls patellar position, are too tight; this results in patellar tilt and subsequent overload of the bone and cartilage of the outer half of the kneecap. Many people respond well to conservative treatment designed to stretch the lateral retinaculum. However, if the conservative treatment is not successful, a lateral release may be needed.

The lateral retinaculum is cut through from the top to the bottom of the kneecap. (The retinaculum is made of similar material to ligaments and is much like a strap or band that holds the other structures in place.) This allows the patella to assume a normal balanced position, which is centered in the trochlear groove. Thin scar tissue forms at the edges of the cauterized ligament sections, eventually filling in the gap created by the surgery. This leaves the retinaculum in a more relaxed state.

After an arthroscopic lateral release, you may need crutches for several days, and physical therapy usually begins shortly after surgery. A return to sports activity takes three months on average.

Proximal and Distal Realignment

Proximal means closest to the point of attachment, and *distal* means farthest from the point of attachment. A proximal realignment corrects the position of a kneecap that subluxes or dislocates laterally—toward the outside of the knee. This may occur as a result of trauma or because you are loose jointed. In this procedure, the soft tissue structures on the inside (medial) retinaculum are tightened to help keep your kneecap properly centered. There is a thickening of this retinaculum, called the medial patellofemoral ligament, which can be repaired or reconstructed at the time of the proximal realignment. Sometimes this is performed in combination with a lateral release to optimally balance the position and tracking of the patella.

A distal realignment is needed if the patella dislocation or subluxation results from an abnormality in the angle of attachment of your patellar tendon. In this case, an osteotomy, or bone cut, is made across the tibial tubercle, the small bump where the patella tendon attaches. The attachment site of the patella tendon is shifted toward the medial to optimize patellar tracking. The tibial tubercle can also be shifted forward to relieve the pain caused by instability and local arthritis. There are a variety of distal procedures designed to treat isolated patellofemoral arthritis by decreasing the load across the patellofemoral joint. In all distal realignment procedures, an osteotomy of the tibial tubercle is performed, with the position of the tubercle shifted to optimize patellar tracking and decrease patellofemoral forces. The osteotomy is secured with two large screws, which remain in place until the osteotomy is healed.

Realignment surgery requires a longer recovery time. Depending on the procedure, the quality of your bone, and stability of the osteotomy fixation, you may be on crutches for two to six weeks and may need a brace for six to twelve weeks. Total time of recovery can range from four to nine months, so it is crucial that you discuss the specific plan for your surgery—and afterward—with your surgeon.

SURGERY FOR INTRA-ARTICULAR FRACTURES

When you fracture the portion of your patella, femur, or tibia that is inside the knee joint, it is called an intra-articular fracture. In most cases of intra-articular fracture, there is a concomitant injury to the articular cartilage. There are two types of intra-articular fractures: open fractures, where the skin is broken; and closed fractures, where the skin and soft tissues around the knee are intact.

Open fractures involving the knee joint or lacerations exposing the knee joint are an emergency, and surgery should be done within six hours of the trauma. This surgery is done to stabilize the damaged parts of the knee and to clean out any debris or damaged tissue present in or around the knee to decrease the risk of an infection developing.

Closed fractures may not be an emergency, but surgery will be required soon if there are significant gaps, or alterations in the normal contours of the articulating surfaces of the femur, tibia, or patella. These procedures are best performed within the first week or two following the trauma. Depending on the type and complexity of the fracture, a combination of arthroscopic and open surgery may be needed.

The recovery from an intra-articular fracture absolutely depends on the type and location of fracture, the amount of joint articular surface involved, the type of fixation (plates, screws), and the quality of your bone. An intra-articular fracture can significantly increase your risk of posttraumatic arthritis and knee stiffness, because of the damage to the articular cartilage. In some cases, these injuries can limit your return to a fully active lifestyle.

BONE CANCER SURGERY

There are many surgical techniques used in treating bone cancer, but before surgery to treat the cancer, a surgical biopsy must be done. This involves removing a piece of the tumor to determine the type, grade, and stage of cancer. It is best that the biopsy and subsequent surgery are planned together and that the same orthopedic surgeon at the cancer center perform both procedures. Whenever possible, surgeons try to remove just the tumor and an area of healthy tissue around it.

WHAT TO EXPECT AFTER KNEE SURGERY

Any surgical procedure, whether arthroscopic or open surgery, as an outpatient or requiring a hospital stay, will impact your daily life. Doctors understand that patients' expectations can play a significant role in how they recover from surgery and how satisfied they are with the results, so it's important to know what to expect.

Managing Pain

There may be significant pain to manage after surgery while your knee heals. Ask your doctor how much pain should be anticipated and how best to manage it. It is easier to manage pain when you take your medications on a regular basis rather than waiting until you feel pain. Many oral pain medications take thirty to forty-five minutes to be absorbed and effective. Pain medications come in many types, ranging from acetaminophen and NSAIDs to mild and potent narcotics. Many narcotic pain medications can make you nauseous, and if you have had bad experiences with any, let your doctor know in advance. People perceive and experience pain very differently, and it helps your doctor to have some idea of how you might respond. Some people are stoic and won't acknowledge pain until it is severe, while others have a much lower threshold.

For an arthroscopic procedure, your doctor may prescribe medications such as NSAIDs and a mild narcotic such as codeine or hydrocodone with acetaminophen. For open surgery, stronger medications such as Percocet may be needed for the first few days. Many hospitals have a pain management program where anesthesiologists and nurse anesthesiologists work with you to control your pain. If you are an inpatient after surgery, a PCA (patient controlled analgesia) pump may be used. You can control the frequency of an intravenous or epidural pain medication within limits set by the anesthesiologist. (See chapter 14 for more information about medication.)

Maintaining Good Circulation

To help diminish swelling of your knee, calf, or foot, sit or lie with your leg elevated at the level of your heart. Your doctor or physical therapist may advise you to move your feet up and down at regular intervals to help blood flow through the calf. You may also be advised to bend and straighten your knee to keep it from getting stiff.

Bearing Weight

Your surgeon may want you to use crutches or a cane for a certain length of time. If you are allowed to bear as much weight as you can comfortably tolerate, then you can gradually put more weight on your leg as discomfort subsides, and you gain strength. For some procedures, such as osteotomy or ACL reconstruction, you may be fitted with a brace to protect your knee while it heals. If your surgeon puts you in a brace, it is for a good reason, so don't discontinue or change the brace without checking first with your doctor. Some cartilage resurfacing procedures or meniscal repairs require the use of modified weight bearing or crutches for up to six weeks after surgery.

Your questions regarding weight bearing, crutches, and braces should be answered *before* surgery so that you can anticipate your needs. If your surgery involves your right knee, your ability to drive may be limited. If your home has a lot of stairs, you need to be prepared for how much you'll be able to move around.

Caring for the Wound

Whether you have arthroscopic or open surgery, the incision will be closed with sutures or surgical staples. Some sutures will dissolve and don't need to be removed. Others will need to be removed in the first or second week following surgery when the wound begins to close. A bandage is applied to your knee after surgery, and your surgeon will tell you when to change or remove it. In some cases, the dressing is removed the day after surgery, but many bandages remain in place for several days. It is very important to keep your bandages dry and clean. Until your sutures are removed, you will not be able to swim or get in a hot tub or bathtub. Some surgeons will permit showering several days after an arthroscopic procedure. For open surgery, the wounds must be kept dry until suture or staple removal. Avoid directing water at the incisions when you shower, or look for some plastic shower bags at a medical supply store. Always follow your surgeon's instructions to avoid complications such as postoperative infection, which can result from poor wound care.

Getting Rehabilitated

Depending on the type of surgery, you will likely need supervised physical therapy to help restore full range of motion, strength, and function to your knee. This usually begins in the hospital and continues after you go home. As you progress, you may have temporary setbacks. If your knee hurts or swells, discuss this with your physical therapist and modify activity until you feel better. If symptoms persist, contact your doctor. (See chapter 13 on physical therapy.)

Avoiding Problems

Postoperative complications may include superficial (skin) or deep (joint) infection, or a blood clot in your calf veins (deep vein thrombosis) or lungs (pulmonary embolus). Precautions are taken to avoid these complications, and they are treatable if they occur. Call your doctor if you have any signs of infection, including fever, chills, redness near or around the incision, increasing tenderness or swelling of the knee, wound drainage, and intensifying knee pain. Your doctor should review these signs with you.

Warning signs of a deep vein thrombosis (DVT) in your calf include increasing pain or swelling in your calf or foot, or tenderness and redness above or below your knee. If you are short of breath, suffer sudden chest pain, or have chest pain and coughing, call 911 and notify your doctor immediately. He or she will send you to an emergency room for evaluation. These symptoms could be signs of a blood clot traveling from your leg to your lungs, which can be fatal if ignored.

If you plan to travel soon after surgery, discuss the trip's timing with your surgeon. It is sometimes appropriate to use medication to decrease the risk of DVT if airline or extended car travel is necessary. If you use oral contraceptives or have a personal or family history of DVT, make sure that your surgeon is aware of this before surgery. This may result in changes in your postoperative medications, treatment, and travel recommendations made by your surgeon.

KEY POINTS

- Surgery is needed if there is an injury or condition that cannot be treated successfully with medication, physical therapy, rest, or avoidance of the provocative activity.
- The majority of sports-related knee surgery is performed using arthroscopy or an arthroscopically assisted technique.
- Minimally invasive open surgery is sometimes

needed for osteotomy, patellar realignment, and cartilage resurfacing such as mosaicplasty and ACI.

- Open repair is indicated for quadriceps or patellar tendon ruptures, patellar fractures, complex fractures involving the knee joint, and partial or total knee replacement surgery.
- Emergency knee surgery is needed for open or penetrating injury to the knee.
- Be sure that you understand your knee problem and the surgical solution to your condition before your surgery, so you can manage your expectations.
- Make a list of questions to ask your surgeon so that you know what to expect before and after surgery.
- Physical therapy before surgery may speed your recovery.
- Simple or extensive physical therapy may follow surgery to restore range of motion and normal function to the knee. The type and duration depends on the surgery performed.

Chapter 16

Knee Replacement Surgery

Frank, a fifty-year-old firefighter, had damaged his knees playing football as a young man and compounded this damage with several injuries on the job. He had had cortisone injections for pain and arthroscopy to smoothe the cartilage surface, but his knees were too far gone for anything but a bilateral knee replacement.

"I used to grind my teeth in my sleep," he said, describing his constant pain. "At work I needed total adrenaline to get through the day. I used to eat Tylenol like candy, taking six to eight a day. Now I can wake up in the morning without pain. I can go up and down stairs. I enjoy walking.

"When I took my first steps without support about six weeks after surgery, I felt like Frankenstein walking. I know I won't ever be fluid or graceful but since my knee replacement surgery, I can turn around normally. Last winter when we had snow and ice, I felt nervous about going out. I fear knocking knees with people or having a

shopping cart bang into me in the market, although each day I get more confident.

Most people who undergo knee replacement surgery experience a dramatic reduction in knee pain and are able to perform daily activities that have caused them pain for years. The majority of knee replacements are performed on people over the age of sixty, but everyone is evaluated individually, based on pain suffered and disability. Knee replacements have been successful with all ages, from young teenagers with juvenile rheumatoid arthritis to older people with degenerative arthritis. The potential complications and long-term success vary according to each individual's condition.

In the early days of knee replacement, prostheses were little more than crude hinges that didn't sufficiently replicate normal anatomy. They had a high failure rate. However, over the last twenty years there have been great advances in design and fit of knee implants. Now, with a 90 percent to 95 percent success rate for knee replacement, your surgeon can choose a prosthesis that takes into account your age, weight, activity level, knee stability, and gender.

Women receive the majority of the approximately half million knee replacements performed in the United States each year—about 63 percent—because they are more likely than men to have osteoarthritis and other damage to their knees late in life. In light of this trend, prostheses that are sized to fit women and men of all sizes are now available. A woman's distal femur, the part farthest from the knee joint, is usually longer from front to back and narrower from side to side than a man's. As a result, the unisex implants of the past were a bit too wide in some women and would over-hang slightly onto soft tissue, especially in smaller women. The implant manufacturers have since responded to this problem by creating implants more geometrically suited to the female knee. Not all women require a gender-specific knee. The decision is based on your bone structure and anatomy, not just your gender. There are many brands of knee prostheses available, but your surgeon will likely have a preference for a particular type based on his or her training and experience. You need to rely on your surgeon to make the decision concerning the type of prosthesis you will need based on your age, activity, and weight.

WHAT PROSTHESES ARE MADE OF AND HOW THEY STAY PUT

Knee replacement joints are made of a combination of a special plastic called high molecular weight polyethylene (UHMWP) and metal (titanium or cobalt-chromium-based alloys). The prosthesis is designed to replicate your knee's natural ability to roll and glide as it bends. The femoral component is a strong, polished piece of metal that curves around the end of your femur. It has an anterior femoral groove where the kneecap can move up and down smoothly as you bend or straighten your knee. The tibial component is a metal platform with a polyethylene cushion or spacer that locks into the metal tray. The patella is a dome-shaped piece of polyethylene with or without a metal backing.

The majority of knee replacements are held in place with fast-curing cement called polymethylmethacrylate (PMMA) which forms a permanent bond between the metal or plastic and the underlying bone. This bond can last for more than twenty years, depending upon your activity level, weight, and general health. When the replacement is implanted without cement, the texture of the implant or a coating applied to it facilitates bone growth directly into the surface of the implant. Screws or pegs may be used to stabilize the implant until the bone growth occurs. By relying on the bone growth, this type of implant takes a longer time to heal and stabilize. It can be just as successful as the cemented type in relieving pain and restoring function, but a porous in-growth prosthesis would be more likely to be used in a younger patient with dense, strong bone than an older patient.

There is also a hybrid design that allows the femoral component to be inserted without cement, and the tibial component with cement. This technique began in the 1980s, so long-term results are just now being measured and are generally positive.

TOTAL KNEE REPLACEMENT

At present, the majority of knee replacements performed in the United States are total knee replacements (TKR). That is, the entire joint is replaced with artificial material. The end of your femur is removed and replaced with a metal shell, or resurfacing cap. The end of your tibia is also removed and replaced with an implant consisting of metal and polyethylene. The back of your kneecap is resurfaced with polyethylene that may or may not have a metal backing.

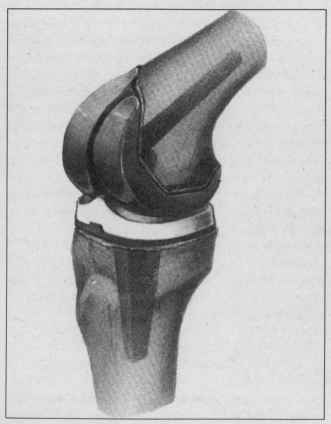

FIGURE 5. A total knee replacement attaches the femur to the tibia. The artificial joint is made of metal and plastic, and is usually held in place with cement as well as screws and pegs. (© *Olga Spiegel, 2007.*)

TKR is appropriate if your knee has been damaged by progressive osteoarthritis, inflammatory arthritis, or trauma, and if two or more compartments (medial, lateral, patello-femoral) are affected. Osteoarthritis is the most common reason for TKR in this country.

The surgical approach to TKR continues to change. In the past, large incisions were used, with extensive stripping of soft tissue structures around the knee. Now surgeons are commonly utilizing smaller incisions to achieve the same goals, resulting in less scarring and trauma to your knee. Not all TKR can be done using these minimally invasive techniques, though. The decision to use such techniques is made based on your weight, knee alignment, and the degree of arthritis or deformity present in your knee.

Total knee replacements do not have the capacity to rejuvenate themselves. They can fail over time if the cement loosens, the polyethylene surfaces wear out, or if the implants become disconnected from the bone.

Even though the metal is polished smooth, and the polyethylene is treated to resist wear, the loads and stresses of daily knee movements can generate microscopic particulate debris. This in turn can trigger the inflammatory response called osteolysis. Inflammatory cells respond to the particulate debris, become activated, and release enzymes that can damage the bone around the prosthesis. This results in what is known as aseptic loosening. Doctors don't yet know why this process is more aggressive in some people than in others, but it is the focus of many scientific studies at academic medical centers around the country.

PARTIAL KNEE REPLACEMENT

Partial, or unicompartmental, knee replacement is not as common as total replacement, but it is appropriate for 6 to 8 of every 100 candidates for knee replacement. *Uni* means "one," so with a unicompartmental replacement, your surgeon will remove only one part of the joint between the tibia and femur. If damage is limited to either the inner (medial) or outer (lateral) part of the knee joint, that part can be replaced without sacrificing the normal portions of the joint. Unicompartmental surgery is best suited for people who are older, thinner, and less active. It requires smaller and less invasive incisions, so there is less trauma to muscles around the knee. As a result, recovery and rehabilitation are typically faster than from a TKR.

BILATERAL KNEE REPLACEMENT

Bilateral knee replacement refers to a TKR performed on both knees. Many people have severe arthritis in both knees and may opt to have bilateral knee replacements done during the same surgery or as staged procedures during a single hospital stay. Others prefer staged procedures that are performed weeks or months apart. If you know that both your knees are candidates for replacement, you will want to discuss the pros and cons of the types of bilateral surgery with your doctor. The decision is based on your medical status, complexity of the knee replacement surgery, and a multitude of lifestyle factors that your surgeon needs to know about. For example, if you must drive a car or truck for your job, then it might be wiser to do one knee at a time. If you have the option of staying at home for a few months after surgery, and you have someone at home to assist you with your chores, then you may be able to have both knees replaced at the same time.

IS KNEE REPLACEMENT RIGHT FOR YOU?

Knee replacement has given a new lease on life to people suffering from injuries, arthritis, and other painful knee problems for years. Knee replacement is generally recommended when less invasive ways to treat your knee condition are no longer working. The decision should be a cooperative one between you and your family, your orthopedist, and your family doctor. This is a highly personal decision based on your pain, activity level, and limitation of lifestyle caused by your knees. Discuss your options for both nonsurgical and surgical treatment before making a decision. Choose your surgeon based on experience and expertise. Ideally, you should seek out a surgeon who performs a minimum of twenty knee replacement surgeries a year. In many communities, excellent TKRs are performed by general orthopedic surgeons, but in a big city you are more likely to see a subspecialist whose practice focuses on joint replacement surgery.

To get an idea if replacement is for you, ask yourself some of these questions:

- Do you have evidence of significant arthritis on X-ray?
- Is your knee pain constant (chronic) even at rest?
- Are daily activities, such as getting up from a chair,

climbing stairs, or walking, limited by your knee pain?

- Do stiffness and swelling prevent you from extending or bending your knee?
- Have you tried other treatments to relieve your symptoms, including medications, braces, physical therapy, and less invasive surgery, without relief of symptoms?
- How old are you? Most knee replacement surgeries are performed in people over the age of fifty because of the potential for component wear. For a younger person, replacement might have to be repeated in later years.
- What do you weigh? If you are significantly overweight, your knee replacement may be prone to early wear.
- Are you in good health? If you have diabetes, vascular disease, or heart disease, you may be at increased risk for complications from surgery. Consulting with your medical doctor can help guide your decision.

GETTING READY FOR KNEE REPLACEMENT

If you are a candidate for knee replacement, you will receive a very comprehensive medical screening. In addition to the primary damage to your knee, your orthopedic surgeon will assess your knee's current range of motion and the muscle strength of your legs. You will also go through a complete physical exam, including a chest X-ray, a checkup with your dentist, blood and urine tests, and an electrocardiogram.

This is the time when you should ask your doctor to describe how the surgery is carried out, what it will accomplish, what to expect afterward, and what needs to be done following surgery to be sure your replacement knee functions properly. Discuss the immediate risks of surgery as well as long-term risks with mechanical knees.

Preoperative Education

Most medical centers that specialize in orthopedic surgery provide a comprehensive education program prior to surgery for people scheduled for joint replacement. A nurse educator will explain what you can expect during the preoperative planning, surgery, recovery, and rehabilitation processes surrounding knee replacement. The class prepares you and your family for surgery and the hospital experience. This approach can especially enhance recovery because it helps you create a plan for functioning at home in the first few weeks with your new knee—a time when you may need a cane, crutches, or a walker to get around. You will need help with everyday tasks such as bathing, cooking, and doing laundry. If you live alone, ask the hospital social worker or the staff in your surgeon's office to help you find someone to assist you, or perhaps to arrange for a short stay in an extended care facility. You will need to arrange for this assistance well before the day of surgery.

Your home should be prepared ahead of time:

- Live on one level. You may not be able to climb stairs easily for a while, so it will be helpful if you can sleep, bathe, and eat on the same level.
- Modify the bathroom. A support bar in your

shower or bathtub is a good idea. Is there a high bench or chair you can install in the shower temporarily? In addition, a support bar may come in handy near the toilet. If you are replacing both knees, consider installing a toilet seat riser with arms to help you get up and down.

- Make your home fall proof. Be sure there are no loose rugs, wires, or other objects in your living space that can trip you. Also, make sure that your furniture is arranged so that you don't bump into sharp table edges or corners.

- Arrange a special place to sit. A comfortable, stable chair will allow you to relax and elevate your leg. The chair should have a firm cushion and back, two arms, and a footstool for intermittent elevation. The seat should be eighteen to twenty inches from the ground.

- Keep everything within easy reach. You don't want to have to use a step stool to reach high cabinet shelves, or get down on your knees to retrieve pots and pans or other supplies. Make sure everything you need—clothing, food, dishes, toiletries, and medical supplies—is within easy reach.

Physical Therapy before Surgery

Having a short course of physical therapy before replacement surgery can make your recovery easier. A physical therapist will guide you through stretching and strengthening of your quadriceps, hamstrings, calf, and hip muscles, so that you will have more strength for using your new knee. Many people have completed a series of physical therapy visits prior to their TKR as part of conservative management. The duration of preop physical therapy is very dependent on your average (baseline) activity level and limitations. People who have badly damaged knees may not have this therapy first.

THE SURGERY

The operating rooms at large orthopedic medical centers have been specially designed for joint replacement procedures. These large rooms have special air control systems to minimize the risk of infection associated with joint replacement surgery. In addition, regional anesthesia and patient controlled analgesia make recovery easier and more comfortable.

Knee replacement surgery is performed through an open incision of six to twelve inches. The length of incision depends on your body type (how muscular you are, how much fat is below the surface of your knee) and the degree of knee deformity. The damaged cartilage and bone are removed, rough edges smoothed, and you are measured for the prosthesis. Your surgeon will attach the prosthesis to the end of your femur and tibia and to the back of your kneecap. Before the incisions are closed, the surgeon bends and rotates the knee to be sure it is functioning properly. It takes one to two hours for a TKR to be completed.

Recovery in the Hospital

After surgery, you will be in the recovery room—postanesthesia care unit (PACU)—until your doctor determines you are ready to go home. Typically, patients stay in the hospital three to five days before going home or to a rehabilitation center.

Managing pain. Always let the nurses and doctors know if you hurt. Many modern medical centers have a dedicated acute pain service. This group of anesthesiologists and nurses will work with you to help manage your pain. Pain medication can be given in multiple forms, from oral to intravenous to epidural. (See chapter 14 on medications.)

Moving your legs. Soon after surgery, you will begin moving your new knee and walking with assistance. You will be asked to move your foot and ankle to optimize blood flow to your leg muscles and to prevent foot and ankle swelling. This also helps prevent blood clots by not letting the blood rest in the leg veins. Wearing support hose or compression boots offers further protection against DVT. While you are in bed, a CPM will slowly bend and straighten your knee to decrease pain and improve knee motion. If you don't feel secure in the device, or your leg is not seated properly, be sure to ask for help.

Physical therapy. The day after surgery, a physical therapist will visit to show you how to exercise your knee safely and will continue to work with you in the following weeks to improve your mobility and strength. By six weeks after surgery, you are likely to be able to give up your cane, drive a car, and return to work. If you have bilateral knee replacements, your recovery time will be longer, but you will only have to go through recovery once instead of twice.

POSSIBLE COMPLICATIONS OF
KNEE REPLACEMENT SURGERY

There is a low complication rate for knee replacement surgery. The most common complication is a blood clot in a leg vein, but your surgeon will help you prevent this with periodic elevation of your legs and exercises for your lower legs to increase circulation. Many surgeons will recommend medication to decrease the risk of a blood clot, such as aspirin or Coumadin. An ultrasound study or venous Doppler is generally performed prior to hospital discharge to see if you have even a small or asymptomatic blood clot in a vein. The presence or absence of a DVT will determine the type and duration of anticoagulant therapy used for the first six weeks following surgery.

Nerve damage is uncommon but can occur if a nerve has been stretched as it passes the knee joint. This may result in areas of numbness or muscle weakness, though it usually improves with time. Nerve damage is more common if correction of a significant knee deformity is needed. Your surgeon will consult with a neurologist to determine how long it will take for the affected nerve to recover.

Internal scarring of the knee may occur following TKR, which can limit motion and cause pain. Your surgeon will monitor your range of motion carefully and may recommend manipulation—a forceful bending of the knee under anesthesia—if you are having trouble regaining your range of motion. Because this method of breaking up the scar tissue can be painful, anesthesia is used.

The biggest worry for you and your doctor is the risk of infection. An infection in the knee occurs in fewer than 2 percent of people undergoing knee replacement surgery. Infection can occur in the days to weeks following surgery, but it can also occur years later. A delayed, or late-onset, infection is caused by bacteria from your bloodstream that infect the knee. For this reason you will need to take antibiotics before having any dental work done or other medical procedures, such as a colonoscopy. Tell your doctor if you develop a fever, chills, swelling, or tenderness in the area of the knee replacement—even years after successful surgery.

A major complication such as a heart attack, pulmonary embolus, or stroke is rare during knee replacement surgery. If you have a chronic illness that could complicate your recovery, it is important to discuss the potential risks with your surgeon and medical doctor. Anyone undergoing major surgery such as TKR will have a thorough evaluation performed by an internist prior to consideration for surgery. You are cared for by both your internist and orthopedic surgeon while in the hospital.

REHABILITATION AFTER KNEE REPLACEMENT SURGERY

Your rehabilitation program will begin while you are in the hospital and will continue after discharge at an outpatient physical therapy center or an inpatient rehabilitation facility. On average, if you have one knee replaced, you might spend one to two weeks in a rehabilitation facility, but in some cases, you may not need it at all. Following a bilateral knee replacement, you may need to spend at least two weeks in rehab, with physical therapy several times a day.

Once you go home, you will need to continue an exercise program until you gain normal knee function. This might involve physical therapy three times a week at a center for as long as several months. How often you attend physical therapy at the center will depend on your age, general health, and goals for recovery. Even if you are quickly feeling normal, don't skip the therapy. Your goal after surgery is to optimize your range of motion, strength, and endurance so that you can begin to enjoy activities previously limited by your painful knees, and consistency is key to a healthy and full recovery from surgery.

Most outpatient physical therapy programs following replacement are held two to three days a week and may include therapeutic massage of your leg and kneecap. Massage can be painful because your therapist will use manual pressure to help diminish internal scar tissue and improve gliding of the soft tissues. After massage and stretching, your knee is treated with ice to relieve the pain and decrease swelling.

Your therapist will create a customized recovery program for you based on your medical condition, your strength before surgery, your range of motion, and postoperative goals. Surgeons and therapists usually work together to design a program, which can have different features for different people.

Going Home

You should follow your surgeon's and therapist's instructions concerning wound care, exercise, and follow-up appointments to check your condition. Walking in your house and then outdoors will gradually increase your mobility as you resume your normal strength and activities. Several times a day, you will need to do the knee strengthening exercises that your therapist has taught you.

Most normal activities such as shopping and household chores are within your reach within three to six weeks after knee replacement. You need muscle control to drive, so it may take time before you can drive safely. Your therapist can help guide you in this decision.

Once fully recovered, you can walk, swim, ride a bike, play golf, and even participate in doubles tennis. However, jogging or running is never recommended, as it may result in premature wear or loosening of your artificial joint. It is very important to discuss your expectations for activity after TKR with your surgeon so that you have a clear understanding of possible restrictions.

Overcoming the Fear of Falling

Anyone with a new knee needs time to adjust and feel confident that he or she can walk around without mishap. This is especially true right after surgery, when your muscular strength has not fully recovered. It can be hazardous to walk up or down stairs without assistance until your knee is strong and mobile. That's why it's important to use a cane or crutches or have someone help you. For some people, a walker is needed to support weight and provide balance. It is crucial to follow your physical therapist's directions to develop strength in the leg muscle, so that you can achieve confidence with balance and body position in space.

Getting Used to Your New Knee

The skin around your knee incision will feel numb or may tingle for months after surgery. The incision will be red and raw looking in the early weeks after your surgery.

However, both the numbness and the appearance of the scar will steadily improve with time.

Your knee replacement will make knee motion easier and less painful. You will be able to go up and down stairs, get in and out of a car, and return to moderate activity. Your knee bending will have limitations that are based on the range of motion of the prosthesis. If you feel some soft clicking of the metal and plastic when you bend or walk, that is normal and will become much less noticeable in the ensuing months.

> **AIRPORT SECURITY TIP**
>
> The amount of metal in your knee will set off airport security devices, so it's a good idea to carry a card from your surgeon documenting your TKR and to let the security agent know about it ahead of time.

KEY POINTS

- Total knee replacement surgery—TKR—now has a 90 percent to 95 percent success rate.
- Bilateral knee replacement can involve having both your knees replaced simultaneously or during separate surgeries.
- Women and older adults receive the majority of knee replacements.
- Physical therapy following knee replacement is critical to achieving success.
- Keep your expectations realistic; there may be some activities, such as jogging, that you will not be able to do after knee replacement.

Chapter 17

Complementary and Alternative Therapy

Complementary or alternative therapies can help manage knee pain, but will not cure your knee pain unless they are used in combination with traditional medical care as part of an integrative treatment program. The term *complementary* medicine implies that these therapies are used to complement or support conventional therapies for pain, while the term *alternative* therapy suggests that these therapies are mutually exclusive.

Complementary and alternative therapies have become more mainstream and are frequently referred to as CAM. Under this umbrella term are chiropractic, acupuncture, massage therapy, homeopathy, and naturopathy, as well as an array of mind-body techniques such as biofeedback and meditation.

Until recently, there was an attitude of "Don't ask, don't tell" in relation to CAM. That is, patients didn't tell their doctors they were using these practices, and doctors failed to ask their patients if they were. Now doctors know this policy is unhelpful. Any complementary technique or herbal supplement that you use should always be shared with your doctor to help prevent bad reactions to the combination of medication and herbal supplements or other practices.

Americans spend approximately $27 billion a year on herbal remedies, chiropractors, and massage therapists. In the 1990s, as the popularity of alternative medicine grew and the cost of traditional medicine soared, the National Institutes of Health began funding studies to provide the public with useful information regarding the effectiveness of these treatments. Scientists discovered, when used wisely, certain treatments can ease symptoms of chronic pain, stress, and anxiety, enhance the effects of conventional medical treatment, and improve your overall mood and outlook.

In general, complementary therapies do not replace conventional therapy, cure illness, or improve an acute condition quickly. The potential for harm from some alternative therapies such as herbal remedies reflects the lack of FDA oversight for many of these remedies and nutritional supplements. Just because something is "all natural" does not mean that it is safe. You need to ensure that the supplement contains the material that is listed on the label and that this material doesn't interact with other medications that you are taking. For example, the herb St. John's Wort, used to help manage minor depression, may result in serious complications during anesthesia for surgery, so you should tell your doctor if you are taking this herbal remedy to avoid serious harm during surgery.

Always let your doctor know about every vitamin, herbal supplement, exercise, or manual manipulative therapy you use. Your doctor may have experience with complementary practitioners and be able to offer recommendations for reputable massage therapists, acupuncturists, or energy healers. In the long run, the role of acupuncture and other nontraditional pain control methods has to be determined through outcome studies. Ask these questions of your alternative or complementary medicine provider before you undertake any therapy:

- How effective is the treatment, and for how long does it last?
- What are the costs and risks?
- How does it compare to other treatments for the same problem?
- May I see your license and credentials?

ACUPUNCTURE

Acupuncture is an ancient Chinese therapeutic process in which specific points of the body are stimulated with needles to foster healing or pain relief. The theory is that the body's energy—*qi* (pronounced *chee*)—is carried along pathways called meridians. When you are ill, the flow of *qi* in the twelve primary meridians of your body is out of sync. For example, rheumatoid arthritis (RA) is a painful inflammatory condition that falls into the realm of interrupting *qi*. Inflammatory conditions reflect an excess of *qi*, while dull pains and stiff joints are indicative of a deficiency. This probably mirrors the evolution of RA from an early stage when it is highly inflammatory to a chronic late state where there is more atrophy, stiffness, and dull aching. The treatment, of course, has to be appropriate for each stage. So the clinician must examine you to determine the stage in order to use the appropriate acupuncture points.

By stimulating specific points along the meridians, it is theorized that the flow can be corrected to optimize health or block pain. Although there is data that acupuncture can be helpful for some conditions, Western researchers tend to believe it does so by stimulating the central nervous system to release chemicals (endorphins) that lessen the *perception* of pain.

A study of acupuncture and knee pain by a team of rheumatologists and licensed acupuncturists at the University of Maryland School of Medicine found that when applied to specific points on the leg, acupuncture can significantly relieve pain and improve function in people with osteoarthritis of the knee. As summarized in their report in the *Annals of Internal Medicine* in 2004, acupuncture can be used safely in combination with other forms of care and can potentially improve the quality of life for those affected with knee pain. This study was supported by the National Center for Complementary and Alternative Medicine and the National Institute of Arthritis and Musculoskeletal and Skin Diseases.

How It Works

Your acupuncturist will insert as few as five or as many as fifteen thin needles at the 360 specific points along the meridians. As the needles are inserted, you may feel a light needle prick, tingling, warmth, or pinching. The needles are left in place twenty minutes, on average, and a course of ten treatments is usually needed to obtain maximum benefit.

Follow-up treatments, usually once every few months, are advised to maintain normal energy balance. Some therapists may twirl the needles or apply electrical current. Pressure is sometimes applied with fingers or with suction applied by placing small heated jars, which form a vacuum, over the points to bring energy to the surface.

Things to Consider

If your acupuncturist is working with your doctor, they should agree on the cause of your problem, and the approach must be planned out. Acupuncture treatment sessions should not be more than two to three days apart; once a week is not enough. The benefits are not cumulative, and you won't see much benefit unless you have five or six treatments. Also, it is a good idea to have something to eat and drink before you go for treatments.

At present, there is not sufficient data on the frequency of a positive response to acupuncture treatments. Acupuncture is a time-consuming procedure and relatively expensive. It is not yet universally covered by medical insurance. The federal Food and Drug Administration estimates that nine to twelve million patients spend as much as $500 million on acupuncture treatments per year. In the year 2000 an estimated twenty thousand licensed acupuncturists were practicing in thirty-four states and the District of Columbia. In 1999 more than three thousand medical doctors trained in acupuncture were practicing in all fifty states.

Acupuncture has a good safety record when it is performed by licensed practitioners using disposable needles. There is a risk of infection if nonsterile needles are used.

Local bleeding may occur, causing bruising, especially for people taking blood thinners such as Coumadin or Lovenox. Aspirin and other NSAIDs also thin your blood with long-term use.

MASSAGE

Therapeutic massage may be prescribed by your orthopedist as part of your rehabilitation following surgery. This is usually targeted at breaking up scar tissue and restoring function to your knee, but you may find massage a good way to relax your leg muscles and relieve pain.

In today's fast-paced but largely sedentary world, spas offering massage have become more and more popular as a means of stress relief. Therapeutic massage is as old as civilization. Hippocrates, the "father of medicine," believed that massage freed nutritive fluids to flow to the body's organs. The Romans took this a step further and made massage part of their healing system. Eastern cultures in India and China have also developed massage techniques, and today we have various massage styles based on both Eastern and Western techniques.

How It Works

Western massage, such as Swedish, is designed to relax tense muscles to improve range of motion, remove stress, and increase energy. Putting pressure on muscles brings a different sensation into the tissues and relieves pain. Chinese and Japanese forms of massage, such as Shiatsu, improve the flow of energy—or *qi*—through the body's energy channels. Pressure on acupuncture points releases blocked *qi* and restores the body's natural balance.

A course of traditional Swedish massage may help alleviate the pain of knee arthritis, according to a study performed at the University of Medicine and Dentistry of New Jersey. This study, published in *Archives of Internal Medicine,* suggested that massage reduced pain in a similar way to rubbing an injured area. The pressure sends sensory stimuli that compete with the pain stimuli. A lead study author, David Katz, MD, suggested that the improvement in pain may be due to several factors. The study treated sixty-eight people with arthritis of the knee with massage therapy twice a week for four weeks, followed by one session a week for four weeks. At the conclusion of the study, participants had less pain, less stiffness, and better knee function. Massage seems to make arthritic knees more limber, which subsequently encourages people to walk more. This benefit remained two months after completion of treatment.

Things to Consider

If you want to investigate massage's effectiveness in managing your knee pain, you should work with a licensed massage therapist (LMT) who uses therapeutic muscle massage to improve musculoskeletal disorders. Massage techniques vary from a light touch to a more vigorous stretching of muscles. Some use more forceful pressure application or deep friction massage that can be painful. Make sure you ask what kind of technique will be used and explain to your massage therapist what you are looking for.

Experienced massage therapists may specialize in certain

areas of body work, so find a practitioner who knows the particulars of your knee condition. Ask your doctor or physical therapist for a recommendation. Contact organizations that certify massage therapists, or your state licensing board, to determine the status of the practitioner you are considering. In addition, gather recommendations from other health professionals and ask your massage therapist for references.

MIND-BODY THERAPIES

Pain is heightened by negative emotions and anxiety, which increase muscle tension and may lead to depression. Improving your emotional state has a beneficial effect on your physical status. Mind-body therapies include biofeedback, relaxation techniques, and meditation. These therapies may increase your sense of self-control and accomplishment, but they don't work for everyone. Investigate the technique that appeals to you, and if one doesn't help, try another. Mind-body therapies require time and effort, but they have few side effects and are generally inexpensive.

The Relaxation Response

Dr. Herbert Benson popularized the relaxation response in his best-selling book of that name. It has been used quite successfully to treat various kinds of pain. People experience the response in various ways, such as a sense of well-being, peace of mind, and feeling at ease with the world. These "feelings" constitute an altered state of consciousness, which slows breathing, lowers blood pressure, relaxes muscles, and changes brain wave activity. This response is the opposite of the fight-or-flight response associated with fear or an emergency situation, including pain. There are a variety of techniques to reach this state, but you need to relax. Often repetition of a word or sound, known as a mantra, helps. Transcendental meditation is one technique for achieving this response.

An important feature of this relaxation response is its prolonged benefit, which can far outlast the actual relaxation exercise. It appears that pain is perceived differently under the influence of this response. Pain impulses are still transmitted (body) but are perceived with less suffering (mind). It is as if the alarm reaction of the mind is somehow conditioned to not respond with the same magnitude when confronted by bodily pain. The relaxation response can provide some relief and sense of mastery over your condition.

There are a variety of ways to produce the relaxation response. Deep breathing exercises can potentially calm the sympathetic nervous system (that which controls some of your vital functions, such as heart rate and blood pressure), reducing pulse and blood pressure, and potentially relaxing tight muscles. If you are relaxed, you are likely to experience less pain than if you are anxious or depressed. Once you learn how to breathe deeply from the abdomen, this type of breathing can assist you in achieving a relaxed state. Place your hand over your abdomen as it rises while you inhale and deflates as you exhale. Keep breathing slowly. If you breathe too rapidly, you may get dizzy and develop cramps in your various muscles. This simple breathing exercise along with other relaxation techniques can be used to help decrease the intensity of the pain.

There are many books available for relaxation techniques

such as progressive muscle relaxation, a technique that contracts muscles and then relaxes them, beginning with the feet and moving up through the body. Relaxation techniques are free of side effects and involve minimal or no expense, but lots of effort on your part to gain the benefit.

Meditation

Meditation reduces tension and helps relieve pain. This is performed by focusing your mind on a thought, a sensation, or a single word or phrase to elicit the benefits of the relaxation response. Over time, silent repetition of a word or phrase changes your consciousness. You need a quiet place to meditate, without distractions, and a sitting posture that is comfortable and stable. Meditation begins with deep breathing, while focusing thoughts on a meaningful word, phrase, or object. Your mind will wander and "chatter," but the trick is sticking with the practice long enough to relax and improve concentration.

Yoga

There are several types of yoga, but all reflect a Hindu philosophy that originated in India. Yoga encompasses certain postures and breathing that are considered a form of meditation and/or exercise. At its core, it is meant to help you achieve spiritual centeredness. Common to most forms of yoga is a way of single-pointed concentration that is developed within a specific body posture. Yoga also has significant physical benefits as a technique to improve strength, balance, and flexibility. The best way to learn yoga is to attend a class led by a qualified teacher, but do keep in mind that some positions may be uncomfortable. If you feel pain in your knee—or elsewhere—alter your position or modify the particular pose so that it is pain free.

Biofeedback

You can learn to control certain bodily activities, to raise or lower your pulse and blood pressure, increase blood supply to an area, and relax or contract muscles. Biofeedback helps you modify autonomic nervous system responses. This is the part of the nervous system that automatically controls your minute-to-minute physiology, such as heartbeat and blood pressure, without your awareness. With the help of a trained technician, you are hooked up to electronic instruments that monitor your state of muscle tension, skin temperature, pulse, or brain wave activity. You can learn to voluntarily control the process, including controlling biofeedback from pain.

The basis for biofeedback includes the relaxation response and the work of B. F. Skinner, who showed the scientific community that animals could be taught to control behavior based on a system of rewards. Biofeedback has been touted to help people relax sore muscles and achieve benefit in the treatment of recurring chronic tension headaches, migraines, and some muscle pain.

PILATES

Pilates, or the Pilates Method, is a fitness system developed by Joseph Pilates in the early part of the twentieth century that has become very popular in recent years. Pilates is used to align the body and mind in a series of movements and breathing exercises to gain strength, balance, and awareness. These days, the Pilates Method is used more frequently for rehabilitation, and many physical therapists are now training in the use of Pilates. The principles are centering, concentrating, control, precision, breathing, and flowing movement. Pilates focuses on the large muscle groups at your body's center—abdomen, lower back, hips, and buttocks—and maintains the philosophy that these muscles are the powerhouse from which all energy begins. Joseph Pilates also believed that sloppy, haphazard movements were the cause of injury, and that muscle control was the ideal. Each movement in the Pilates Method has a purpose and is an important part of the whole. No movements are isolated or static. Bone density and joint health are said to improve with practicing Pilates.

While the Pilates Method has teachers and proponents all over the world, if you go to a class at a spa, health club, or gym, make sure you find out about the credentials of the person teaching the course. And here, too, as in yoga and other practices that require certain body positions, if it makes your knee hurt, stop immediately.

TAI CHI

The slow, graceful movements of tai chi increase flexibility and improve balance and coordination, especially in older people. Tai chi is particularly useful for people recovering from chemotherapy-induced fatigue. It is not the same as strength training, in that it doesn't make your muscles stronger. The goal of tai chi is to return the body and mind to their original pure and healthy state. It has been described as a form of "meditation in motion" where the continuity of its movements, combined with the devotion of one's undivided attention, heal and revitalize both the body and mind.

The physical component of tai chi consists of movements aimed at balance, such as correcting angles, squaring hips, controlling the step and the transfer of weight, turning constantly in spirals, opening and closing, centering the trunk, and stretching and relaxing the spine. The movements are gentle, continuous, and circular.

Many find the massagelike movements of tai chi to be effective therapy for a wide range of health problems. The extra degree of stretching and turning in each movement improves health. With practice, these movements affect all body systems. Tai chi can reduce body fat, raising the possibility that it may prevent heart disease. It is one of the few exercises that is appropriate for anybody, regardless of condition. It can even be done in a bed or chair. Tai chi is particularly useful for the frail elderly because it improves balance and flexibility, thus reducing the risk of falls and subsequent fractures common in this age group. It may also help slow bone loss typical in older, inactive people.

KEY POINTS

- Complementary and alternative medicine can be helpful in combination with traditional medical treatment.
- Acupuncture has been used successfully to relieve knee pain from arthritis.

- Massage can be very helpful in easing knee pain and stiffness.
- Relaxation techniques such as meditation, yoga, and Pilates can help you reduce the severity of knee pain by altering your perception of pain.
- Biofeedback can help you to manage knee pain by changing your response to pain signals.
- Tai chi is a good way to develop flexibility and balance.

PART IV

PREVENTION

Chapter 18

Physical Conditioning to Help Your Knees

Ellen and Jim, a retired couple in their eighties, played golf in good weather and in general took long walks. They had always been active and were in excellent condition. They liked to keep up their exercise program, but winter made getting out difficult, so they made a daily early morning trip to their nearby mall, where a local walking club had permission to enter the mall before official opening time. Ellen walked fast, making several complete loops around the mall that amounted to about a mile. Jim, on the other hand, was often distracted and would slow down and look in store windows or talk to some of the others in the group. It isn't hard to guess whose legs were in better shape.

The best way to remain strong and fit is to make exercise a part of your daily life. It is easier to maintain strong and fit muscles than to have to start from scratch, but it is never too late to start exercising. Your muscles may be sore and stiff after the first exercise of the season, but gradually your muscles will acclimate.

Weak muscles play a role in knee injury, so it makes sense to build up your hip, thigh, and calf muscles to support your knees. Balance and stability training also helps the muscles around your knees work together more effectively. Muscle flexibility and strength are crucial to avoiding and relieving knee pain, and many people are able to remain functional with a good exercise program.

Everyone can exercise in some way. For example, leg muscles are strengthened by walking on a level surface, up stairs or hills, by riding a stationary bike, or rowing on an ergometer (a training machine for rowers). Stretching a hamstring can be as simple as putting your leg straight out from your desk chair and leaning toward your toes. If you are new to exercise, it is important to get guidance, start slowly, and gradually develop an exercise program. If you have medical conditions such as high blood pressure, heart disease, or lung disease, consult your physician before beginning an exercise program.

Muscles are designed to work hard, and they do this by contracting and relaxing. When a muscle shortens (contracts), this is called concentric contraction. An example of this is the way your quadriceps works as you straighten your leg when rising from a chair. Muscles can also lengthen as they contract. This is called eccentric contraction. An example of this is the firing of your quad to support your knee as you descend a flight of stairs.

When our muscles work through movement or exercise, they require oxygen to utilize glucose (fuel). If you are performing intense exercise (anaerobic) such as sprinting, the muscle uses a different biochemical pathway to generate energy. This results in lactic acid accumulating in the muscles. The lactic acid is responsible for the burning pain at the end of intense exercise.

The key to effective exercise is to make your muscles more efficient without damaging muscle cells. Intense weight training can result in transient overload injury to muscle, which is often felt one to two days after a very intense bout of strength training. While this is not dangerous, it can take longer for the muscles to heal and may discourage you from exercising, thus defeating your purpose. Finding the appropriate balance between stressing your muscles without causing damage can be difficult for people who are becoming active in sports for the first time in a while. Once you are exercising on a regular basis, you will begin to understand the response of your body to certain types of training. Remember, what works for your friend or training partner may not be right for you. The principles of a good strength training program are these:

- Warm up with five to ten minutes of low-level cardiovascular activity like walking, cycling, or using an elliptical trainer.
- Stretch lightly at the beginning and end of your workout to improve overall flexibility.
- Learn and practice good lifting technique.
- Use proper equipment that is well maintained and in good condition.
- Make certain that the equipment is adjusted for your size. This is especially important for smaller women.
- Make sure you have supportive athletic shoes that fit properly, even for walking.

- Develop a strength training routine so that you will have the necessary muscle strength for your chosen activities.
- Avoid sudden changes in the intensity of exercise.
- Increase the force or duration of activity gradually.
- If you are an athlete, use movement patterns to mimic your sports activity.

Before beginning any type of exercise program, consult your doctor if you have any medical or orthopedic conditions. If you have been treated for an orthopedic condition by a physical therapist, you should review your new program with him or her. It is important to learn how to do your strength/flexibility exercises correctly and to understand which exercises are appropriate for you. Doing the wrong exercise or doing the right ones improperly can lead to injury. Many gyms have training staff who can outline an exercise program for you. A health-care professional can also advise you on how to warm up safely.

KNEE-FRIENDLY AEROBIC EXERCISES FOR ENDURANCE AND STAMINA

Aerobic exercise helps you build muscle endurance and cardiovascular fitness. If you do it regularly, you will notice that you feel more comfortable doing the exercise for increasing amounts of time. Aerobic exercises that are most helpful for people with knee pain are walking, swimming, riding a stationary bicycle, and using an elliptical trainer. Before your knee pain began, you may have been running instead of walking, or doing step classes instead of low-impact aerobics. A step class at your local sports club could be a great aerobic workout, but it might not be very good for your knees. Instead, choose an exercise program that you will continue over an extended period of time, that is easily accessible, and that doesn't cause knee pain.

STRETCHING TO IMPROVE FLEXIBILITY

Stretching is critical to increasing flexibility of your muscles, reducing your risk of injury during exercise or everyday activities, and promoting healthy healing from an injury, yet it is the most neglected component of almost everyone's exercise routine.

Initially, stretching is important because it warms up the muscles and readies the body for exercise. It is also important to stretch *after* you exercise or are active, to ease the tension in your muscles.

Maintaining a flexibility program is important as you age to diminish the stiffness and loss of flexibility that can occur with aging. As you get older, your muscles, tendons, and joints begin to lose some of their natural flexibility. As a result, stretching becomes even more important to maintain fluid movement and range of motion. If you do a light cardiovascular warm-up, such as walking a few blocks before stretching, your muscles will be more pliable and may respond better to flexibility training. Do stretches that involve the muscles you most commonly use in your work or sports activities, as well as the muscles that support your knees: the hamstrings, quadriceps, calves, and hip muscles. Ask your physician, physical therapist, or sports trainer to guide you in stretches that are most suitable for you.

A stretch requires holding a position so that you feel muscle tension but not pain. As you feel the muscle release, you can lean further into the stretch to promote even greater flexibility gains. For example, if you bend over to touch your toes, you might only be able to reach your knees. As you continue to stretch, you might reach your shins and *eventually* your toes! A stretch should be static—that is, slow and steady, and it should be held for about fifteen to twenty seconds. Count out each second, and repeat the stretch up to five times. Do all the stretches slowly until a good feeling develops. You should not feel pain, only the stretch.

In addition to stretching, you can promote flexibility by participating in activities that require and encourage a full range of motion such as yoga, tai chi, Pilates, and various forms of dance. If you are stuck in the same posture all day in your job (sitting or standing), make an effort to periodically change your body position. Move around and stretch in the direction opposite to the position that you sit in. Extend your back and arms, stretch overhead.

Stretching Exercises

Here are some good stretches that are useful for women and men of all ages.

1. Hamstring stretch. Prop your leg on a bench or stair. Stand tall, with your chest high and tummy tight. (Don't let your back collapse inward or bend. If you do you will be stretching your back and not your hamstrings.) Bend forward at the hip, keeping the knee and back straight so you feel the

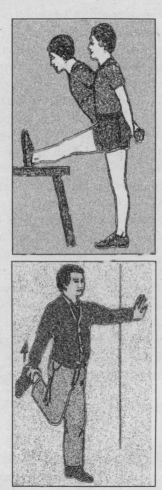

Figure 6. The hamstring stretch (*top*) and quadriceps stretch (*bottom*) keep the muscles that control your knee flexible and help you maintain good range of motion. (© *Olga Spiegel, 2007.*)

stretch behind your thigh and knee. Hold for thirty seconds; repeat one to three times on each side. You can also do this stretch seated in a chair. Stretch your leg out straight, attempt to touch your toes with your fingers, but keep your back flat. Hold this position for a count of thirty and repeat five times.

2. Quadriceps stretch. Stand with one hand on the wall or on the back of a chair. Grasp your ankle with your other hand. Pull your bent leg backward, keeping your knees parallel. Tuck your buttocks under and keep your tummy tight. Bring your heel closer to your buttocks to increase the tension of the stretch. Do not lean forward or allow your back to arch. Hold for thirty seconds and repeat one to three times on each side.

3. Calf stretch. Stand about one arm's distance from a wall. Place both hands on the wall and move one foot forward, so the calf on the other leg stretches. Point your toes directly toward the wall and hold your heels down. Lean into the wall so you feel the stretch in your calf. Hold for thirty seconds and repeat on each side.

4. Gluteus stretch. Stand and prop your bent leg on a table or other solid object. Lean your upper body forward so that you feel a stretch in your buttocks and thigh. Hold for thirty seconds and repeat one to three times on each side.

5. Hip flexor stretch: Stand with your back straight and your knee flexed. With one hand, hold onto a chair or counter to help you balance. With the other hand, reach back and grab your foot and pull

it back away from your body. Hold this position
for a count of ten, then return to the starting
position. You should feel the stretch in the front
of your thigh and the front of your hip.

STRENGTH TRAINING

You can increase your quadriceps strength within several
weeks, even if you are elderly. Increased muscle strength reduces arthritis pain. Once you have your thighs in shape,
you may find some other forms of exercise more fun and
can strengthen your whole body with walking, swimming,
dancing, and low-impact aerobics.

While your main concern should be building up strength
in your hamstrings and quadriceps, calves, and hips so that
you can better protect your knees from injury and damage,
it's a good idea to strengthen other parts of your body as
well. Otherwise, you will have super strong legs but a weak
back. Your back and abdominal muscles will work in tan-
dem with your legs. A strong abdomen and low back are
critical for good posture and balance. Remember, from
head to toe, your body is interconnected, so a weakness in
any one area will affect your overall performance.

Which Type of Strength Training Is Best for You?

There are potential advantages and disadvantages to all
types of strength training. It can be done with exercise machines, resistance bands, calisthenics, or free weights. The
method you choose will depend on your goals, experience,
and the equipment available to you.

- Exercise machines can provide a safe workout for the beginner or experienced athlete but must be adjusted to fit each person. They are useful for muscle isolation. For example, the leg extension machine isolates the quads, while the leg press uses the quads, hamstrings, hip, and calf muscles in concert.
- Resistance bands can be adapted easily to your muscle's need for increased resistance as you become stronger. You can increase the tension of the band by standing farther away from the anchor point.
- Calisthenics are movements that mimic everyday or sports movements. They make the most sense for building practical strength. For example, multiple-joint exercises that involve pushing, pulling, and squatting will provide crossover benefit for many activities and train your muscles the way they will be used. Examples of this are wall squats, jumping rope, or step-ups. You can make this exercise more challenging by stepping up and down on a step while holding a weight in your hands.
- Weights can add more of a challenge to your workout once your strengthening exercises have become easy to do.

It is essential to achieve balance. If you strengthen the muscles in your quads, don't neglect your hamstrings and hips. Exercises for the same body part can be steadily increased by repetition to optimize endurance, or you can increase the weight or resistance while maintaining strength gains and promoting muscular balance.

Strengthening Exercises

1. Leg lift. Lie flat on your back with your left leg
   bent and right leg straight out. Contract your
   quadriceps by lifting your right leg six to eight
   inches off floor or bench; hold for five seconds.
   Keep your thigh muscles tight and lower back
   pressed to floor. Return to the start and repeat. Do
   three sets of ten to fifteen, then repeat on the other
   side. As you develop more strength, you may want
   to add ankle weights. These come with a series of
   one-pound weights that can be added over time
   to ankle straps.

2. Seated leg lift. Sit up straight in a chair with your
   feet shoulder-width apart. Place a folded towel
   under your knees so your toes just brush the floor.
   Slowly raise one foot until your leg is straight in
   front of you with your toes gently pointed back
   toward your body. Pause for a breath as you
   tighten and then release your thigh muscle. Then
   slowly lower your leg to the floor. Do this five
   times for each leg. Over a period of weeks, build
   up to three groups of twenty repetitions each
   on both legs. This exercise may hurt if you have
   patellofemoral pain. If it does, stick to the straight
   leg raises.

3. Hip abduction. Lie on your right side with your
   torso propped up on your right forearm. Make
   sure your right elbow is aligned directly under
   your right shoulder. You may keep your right leg
   straight or bend it for stability. Keeping your left
   leg straight and your knee facing forward, raise

your leg sideways up toward ceiling. Do not allow your left hip to roll forward. Return to start; repeat ten times total. Change sides and repeat using the other leg. You can also do this lying on your abdomen to strengthen the gluteus and hamstring muscles.

4. Tree pose for balance. Stand with your feet shoulder-width apart. Bring your right foot up to rest slightly above or below your left knee. Inhale and reach your arms up. Hold and focus on keeping your balance. Return to start. Switch legs and repeat. Hold this pose for one to two minutes between your other moves. It may look simple, but you're working on balance and strengthening all the muscles around the knee.

5. Minisquats. Stand with your back against wall, then slide down to a near-sitting position. With practice and repetition, slide down to a full sitting position. Be sure to stand on a nonskid surface and keep your feet in front of your knees. You should be able to look down and see your feet. If you can't see your toes, move your feet farther away from the wall. Hold for ten seconds. Repeat ten times at first and eventually work up to thirty reps. If this exercise is painful, try sliding down a shorter distance. The goal is to feel the muscles in your thigh working, not to provoke pain.

Be sure to check with your doctor before you do any of these exercises.

BEST FITNESS EQUIPMENT FOR KNEES

You may have access to a variety of fitness machines at your local health club, physical therapy clinic, or your home. Machines that improve fitness and leg strength include the rowing machine, cross-country ski machine, elliptical trainer, stationary bicycle, and treadmill.

Yoga and Pilates training can be done at home or in a supervised class. It is always helpful to take a series of classes to become familiar with the dos and don'ts before embarking on a home program. There are many fitness tapes, CDs, and TV programs that demonstrate good technique for home use.

THE SPORTS MOST AND LEAST LIKELY TO HURT YOUR KNEES

If you love playing basketball or skiing, there's no reason to stop these activities unless your knees are seriously damaged. With proper training and warming up, you should be able to continue your sport of choice. However, if your knee pain is of concern, you may want to think twice about participating in the sports that are most likely to cause injury.

The National Athletic Trainers' Association (NATA) conducted a three-year study of injuries in high school sports. During the study of 250 schools, 23,566 injuries occurred, and an average of 6,000 students were injured at least once each year. Football had the highest rate of injury, and volleyball the lowest.

In the category of girls' sports, researchers discovered that most injuries occurred during practice rather than during an actual game, with the exception of soccer, which had a larger proportion of injuries in games than practice for both men and women. It may be that athletes spend more time in practice than in an actual game; thus the greater chance of injury.

The knee figures prominently in this survey. Of all the injuries requiring surgery, 60.3 percent were to the knee and occurred during girls' basketball and soccer. While basketball and soccer continue to generate the most injuries in women's team sports, in nonteam sports, skiing leads the list for traumatic injury, and running and tennis for overuse injury.

Many people are highly active but don't call themselves athletes. Rowing is a wonderful sport for people with and without sports experience. The important thing is to learn proper stroke mechanics whether you are training on a rowing ergometer or rowing in a boat. Rowing provides fantastic cardiovascular exercise and is often suitable for people who have sustained knee injuries that make running, soccer, and basketball difficult to continue. The most common injuries seen in rowing are overuse injuries to the patella, shoulder, and low back. Cycling, walking, and swimming are also excellent sports activities for people with knee problems. If you enjoy the competition and camaraderie of team sports, but your knees won't let you play soccer or basketball, you might consider tennis or golf.

CONDITIONING FOR YOUR SPORT

Running and skiing are very common sports among our maturing population. If you enjoy either one or both, it's important that you keep yourself in proper condition so you avoid injury to your knees.

If You Are a Runner

Runners usually stretch their calves, quadriceps, and hamstrings before a run, but you should stretch your iliotibial band as well.

1. Sit on the floor with both legs straight. Cross the leg to be stretched over the straight leg, with the foot placed on the ground. Hold the knee with the opposite hand and pull your body across so that the opposite shoulder touches the stretched leg's knee. Hold for thirty seconds and repeat five times.
2. Stand and prop your leg on a bench or step, with your knee straight. Bend forward at your hip, keeping your back straight so that a stretch is felt in back of your thigh. Hold thirty seconds and do three repetitions.
3. Lie on your back and pull your knee toward your chest. Keep the opposite leg straight. Now straighten your leg slowly, keeping your knee to your chest. Feel the stretch in the back of your thigh, close to your buttock. Hold thirty seconds and do three reps.
4. Stand grasping your ankle with your hand (or a strap). Tuck your buttocks so your back doesn't arch. Bend your knee, keeping your thighs together. Do not rotate your leg in or out and do not bend forward. Pull your heel toward your buttocks to feel a stretch in the front of your thigh.

To stretch the front of your hip, pull your thigh back farther. Then, if you need more of a stretch, bring your heel closer to your buttock. As you bend your knee, make sure your thigh stays in line with your body. Hold thirty seconds and do three reps.

5. With one knee on the floor, lean your whole body forward, keeping your chest upright. Do not allow your front knee to go past your toes. Feel this stretch in front of your rear thigh, close to your hip. Hold for thirty seconds and do three reps.

6. Stand with a wide stance. Shift your weight to one leg by bending that knee. Feel a stretch on the inside of the opposite thigh. Hold for thirty seconds and do three reps.

7. Stand sideways to the wall, with your leg to be stretched away from the wall. Cross your outside leg behind your other leg and toward the wall, making sure that your stance is as wide as possible. Rotate your rear foot slightly outward (away from the wall) and tighten your buttocks. Lean your hips away from the wall and tilt your shoulders toward the wall until you feel a stretch on the outside of your hip. Hold thirty seconds and do three reps.

8. Lie on your back with your knee bent. Use the opposite hand to pull the outside of your knee toward your opposite shoulder. Hold thirty seconds and do three reps.

9. Stand propping your leg straight out on a solid object such as a table. Lean your body forward so that you feel a stretch in the outside of your hip

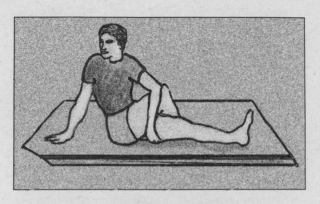

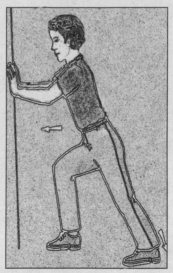

FIGURE 7. Good stretches for runners include the iliotibial band stretch (*top*) and the calf stretch (*bottom*). It is important to stretch before *and after* running or other sports activities. (© *Olga Spiegel, 2007.*)

and buttocks. Hold thirty seconds and do three reps. (You can also do this lying on your back. Position your leg and cross your opposite knee. Then reach behind your opposite thigh and pull your knee toward your chest to get more of a stretch.)

10. Position your body against a wall with one knee bent and the other leg stretched out behind you. Point your toes directly toward the wall and keep your heel down. Lean into the wall, keeping your back knee straight, so that you feel a stretch in your calf. Hold thirty seconds and do three reps.

If You Ski

Conditioning for skiing actually includes all the exercises you need to strengthen the muscles that support your knees. This includes your quads, hamstrings, gluteal muscles (buttocks), hip abductors and adductors (outer and inner hip and thigh), abdominals, back extensors, and the muscles on the inside and outside of your foot and ankle. Here are some types of exercise that amateur skiers practice:

1. Various types of squats, such as those using free weights, your own body weight, and the leg press machine.
2. Standing lunges (both forward and diagonal). If lunges cause knee pain, discontinue this exercise or have a therapist review your technique.
3. Balance exercises, including standing on one leg with the knee slightly bent while moving the other leg in and out, back and forth; standing in ski

position with the knees flexed and shifting your weight from side to side; balancing for a while on each leg.

4. Side-to-side steps, hops, or jumps, with an elastic band and waist belt to increase resistance.

5. Standing or lying leg lifts (out to the side and backward). Keep your stomach tight and move from your hips, not your waist. Or try a hip abductor/adductor machine at the gym.

6. Calf raises by standing with your toes on the edge of a step.

7. Sit-ups and other exercises for upper and lower abdominal muscles; the core of your body.

8. Back extensions such as lying on your stomach and lifting your shoulders. Always get proper directions for such exercises from a sports trainer or physical therapist, because performing any of these movements improperly can injure you.

BEAT THE BARRIERS TO EXERCISE

Good habits are not always easy to start, just as bad habits are hard to break. Failure to exercise regularly is a bad habit. There are a million reasons not to exercise: You are too tired. You have too much to do. You're exhausted after work or child care. Not doing exercise is a habit—a tough one to break. Most people have good intentions but fail to plan for exercise. You have to make exercise an important part of your life, just like going to work, taking care of your family, or doing the chores. Most people plan ahead for vacations because they may have only a certain amount of time. They plan ahead for the menu for an upcoming dinner party. If you are not including regular exercise in your lifestyle, then it's time to apply your problem-solving skills to your personal health and fitness. Here are some suggestions:

There Is No Time

- Wake up earlier and exercise first thing in the morning. Other activities are less likely to get in the way.
- Go for a short, brisk walk on your lunch break.
- Get off your subway or bus stop several blocks early and walk, to combine your commute with exercise.
- Combine activities: have "walking meetings" with business colleagues; walk on the treadmill while watching television.
- Delegate sharing the workload with your spouse and children. Think of it as your duty to teach responsibility, teamwork, and a strong work ethic to your loved ones.
- Prioritize so that errands and work don't sidetrack you. You'll get more done after you are energized with exercise anyway!

You Are Too Tired

- Exercise as early in the day as possible. As the day rolls on, mental fatigue makes it easier to talk yourself out of it.
- Recruit an exercise buddy. The two of you can keep each other going. You will be less likely to miss your

exercise if you know you are letting someone else down.

- Don't stay up late watching television. Turn off the tube and get your sleep.
- Modify your intake of high-sugar foods. They give you a quick high, followed by a real low.
- If you are planning on exercising after work, have a late afternoon snack, such as a nutritional power bar, to give you energy.
- Find activities you enjoy or which provide you with the stress release, stimulation, or social time you need. You'll look forward to being more active.

The Weather Is Bad

- Choose appropriate exercise clothes. The right choices can keep you warm and dry in the cold, and cool in the heat. High-tech fabrics and new garment designs make it easier to handle weather extremes.
- Find indoor options: fitness club, home equipment, exercise videos, or TV shows.
- Walk around the shopping mall, but leave your wallet at home! Many malls have daily walking clubs.
- If nothing else, stretch or do some abdominal strengthening exercises while watching TV.

Who Will Watch the Kids?

- Working moms and dads generally have better success if they exercise during lunch or around the workday when child care is already in place.
- Do a babysitting exchange with neighborhood parents. One of you watches the kids while the others go for a walk or play tennis.
- If you work at home, consider starting or joining a parent-child exercise group.
- Teach your kids to enjoy physical activity by doing it with them: street games, bicycling, hiking, and so on.
- Swap workout time with your spouse.
- Choose at-home options that could be done when kids are napping: yoga, fitness video, indoor bicycle, or treadmill.

EAT WELL AND REDUCE STRESS

One of the most important things your muscles need is water. A big factor in muscle fatigue is not drinking enough water. You need a minimum of eight glasses of nonalcoholic, noncaffeinated beverages daily.

In addition, if you don't get enough protein and complex carbohydrates in your daily diet, then your muscles won't get enough glycogen. Glycogen is the fuel used by your muscles during exercise. Inadequate fuel will result in muscle fatigue and may slow down muscle repair. If you don't get enough nutrients, you also leave yourself open to infections and other illness. Make sure your daily calorie intake matches your need for energy.

When the stress in your life exceeds your ability to cope with it, your body may begin to break down. Knee pain, or any pain for that matter, can be worse when you are stressed and/or depressed. Try to seek professional help to work through emotional issues related to your job, family, social life, finances, and so forth. One of the positive ways to reduce stress is with exercise, so it is important to find a pain-free exercise for your knees and find the time to do it!

KEY POINTS

- A few months of conditioning can help your muscles get strong at any age.
- Stretching is critical to increasing flexibility of your muscles and reducing risk of injury, yet most people who exercise avoid it.
- Weak muscles play a significant role in knee injuries.
- You can reduce arthritis pain by increasing your quadriceps strength even if you are elderly.
- The aerobic exercises that are most helpful if you have knee pain are walking, swimming, riding a stationary bicycle, and using an elliptical trainer.
- Basketball and soccer generate the most injuries in women's team sports. In nonteam sports, skiing, running, and tennis lead the list.
- Good habits are not always easy to start, just as bad habits are hard to break. Failure to exercise is a bad habit.

- A big factor in muscle fatigue is not drinking enough water.
- You need sufficient protein and complex carbohydrates in your diet to fuel your muscles.
- Knee pain is worse when you are stressed or depressed.

Chapter 19

Twenty Ways to Be Good to Your Knees

The idea of prevention is finally taking hold in the American psyche. People are giving up smoking despite continued encouragement from the tobacco companies to counteract that attempt. Fast food chains are offering salads and lower fat menu items, along with their super-sized portions of fat and carbohydrates. Businesses are installing gyms for their employees, offering incentives to stay fit, and beginning walking or group exercise programs. Many health insurance plans will now provide screenings to help identify diseases early enough to provide optimal treatment and prevent disability, and some plans even offer compensation for regular gym attendance.

The way that you treat your knees and your body every day is just as important as the medical treatment provided by your doctor and physical therapist. This book is designed to educate you about the anatomy and physiology of your knees and to describe the cause and treatment of knee pain. But you play an important role in the daily health of your knees. You could be making your knee pain worse at work or play, and with the body weight your knees must support. Even though we now have the technology to replace severely damaged knees, it is easier—and much less expensive—to keep the ones you have.

Make your lifestyle knee-friendly. Common sense and moderation are the most important ingredients in any program designed to maintain healthy knees and to prevent knee pain. Many people active in their younger years want to continue in sports that may no longer be appropriate if their knees have been injured or if they have developed arthritis. At ages fifteen to twenty they can get away with intermittent training for sports, but as they age, maintenance becomes more important.

Competitive contact sports such as football, basketball, and soccer have an increased risk of injury for people of all ages. These sports are fun and can be psychologically and physically rewarding but do carry the risk of injury. There are also occupations that expose your knees to risk of injury that involve repetitive lifting, squatting, and crawling.

1. **Watch Your Weight**
    Many Americans are overweight, a problem that is related to calorie-laden fast foods, gargantuan portions, and lack of exercise. The increase in obesity has been happening gradually over the past few decades because people not only eat more but move less. Americans used to eat three meals a day and do more physical work. Now, they have the opportunity to eat all the time, not only at home, but in the shopping mall, at the movies, the ball

game, and the office breakroom. Work has become less physical, and more hours are spent in sedentary activities.

Being overweight can become a chronic disease from which it becomes more and more difficult to recover. It contributes to the onset of many medical problems, including arthritis, heart disease, diabetes, and cancer. Excess weight can overload your musculoskeletal system and cause premature wear of knee cartilage. Even a modest weight loss can reduce your knee pain.

For most people, the body mass index (BMI) is a good measure to assess whether or not you are overweight. Guidelines from the National Institutes of Health define overweight with a BMI greater than 25. Obesity starts at a BMI of 30. If you are six feet tall and weigh 200 pounds, your BMI is 27, which is a bit high. You would be better off weighing 170 or 180. There is a complicated mathematical formula for calculating your BMI, but it is simpler to go to the National Institutes of Health website and look it up: www.win.niddk.nih.gov/publications/health_ risks.htm#table.

If you are very muscular, your BMI may be elevated even though you are not overly fat. If you are light in weight but have a high body fat, your BMI may appear better than your body actually is. The BMI is not an absolute measure of the "right weight" for you, but it can be used as a guideline you should discuss with your doctor.

2. **Don't Smoke**

   Your lungs are not the only part of your body
   damaged by smoking. All the tissues of your
   body need oxygen to maintain their function, and
   smoking robs these tissues of the optimal amount
   of oxygen. Smoking also increases the risk of
   complications following knee surgery and can
   dramatically slow the healing of bone fractures.

3. **Always Wear Your Seat Belt**

   Crashing into the dashboard of a car during
   an accident is the number one cause of knee
   fractures. This dashboard trauma can also injure
   the articular cartilage in your patellofemoral
   joint and result in injury to the posterior
   cruciate ligament (PCL).

4. **Don't Stand Still**

   Standing still is more tiring than walking.
   Standing in one position for a length of time
   makes the muscles in your lower back tired and
   your knees ache. You may have experienced this
   feeling at a cocktail party, or in a museum or
   shopping center. If you stand for extended periods
   of time, shift from side to side to avoid knee pain.
   If you work behind a counter, keep a step stool
   nearby and alternate raising one leg at a time onto
   the stool periodically. Transfer weight from foot
   to foot, and rock up and down from your heels to
   your toes. These activities take pressure off the
   muscles and the curve of your back. Do this any

time you stand for a prolonged period. Wear supportive, well-cushioned shoes if you need to stand all day.

5. **Don't Sit Still**

Couch potatoes and computer lovers beware: Although modern life has evolved to make you more sedentary, your body has not adjusted to the change. Humans were not designed to sit for extended periods of time. Get up and move periodically. When you sit, use a chair that offers back support—and knee support. This means that the seat length should support your entire thigh. The height of the seat should allow you to place your feet flat on the floor with your knees slightly higher than your hips. Chairs used in offices have an adjustable back and wheels, and the tension and position of the back support should be adjustable along with the height of the seat.

Get up once or change your leg position intermittently. If you are so engrossed in your work that you can't remember, then set an egg timer for thirty minutes so you remember to get up and stretch. Roll your head around to stretch your neck. Lift your arms into the air and stretch. Put your hands on your hips and bend your body forward, backward, and side to side. Do some easy leg stretches.

Bus, truck, and cab drivers also sit for long periods. Anyone seated behind the wheel for long periods should stop every hour or so and walk around. If you cannot do this, change your seat position to alter the angle of your knees. Swing your arms wide and get blood circulating again to avoid stiffness. Lean against the car (or bus) and do some calf stretches. This is especially important if you are still recovering from knee surgery.

6. **Wear Proper Shoes**
   Thank goodness there's no more foot binding, but there are still women who wear shoes that are too pointy-toed and too high, with soles that don't bend or that are too flexible. Avoid flip-flops, high heels, or very flat shoes if you have a lot of walking or standing to do, as most do not provide adequate arch support.

   Careful attention to shoe fit helps avoid injuries and minimizes forces that complicate foot problems. If your shoes don't fit properly, or if they hurt your feet, they will eventually have an effect on your knees.

   Wear the footwear designed for your activity. For example, running shoes are not designed for pivots and turns, but tennis and racquetball shoes are. If you are walking on unpaved paths in the countryside or on cobblestone streets, you may want a walking shoe with good lateral support or even a lightweight hiking shoe. Athletic footwear used to be designed for men, with women's shoes scaled down. But the female foot has a different shape, with a narrower heel compared to the forefoot. Modern sports footwear is better designed to fit the female foot with a wider toe box relative to the heel. There is a lot of variability in sizing and support in athletic shoes, so it is important to try on different brands and styles to find the right shoe for your foot. Be certain that your athletic shoes provide the support and comfort that you need.

Don't run in worn-out running shoes. Train in a supportive, well fitting pair of running shoes with ample room in the toe box. Depending on your weight and running surface, you may need to replace your running shoes every 250 to 300 miles. The sole of your shoe is made with extremely durable rubber, which may still look good even if the midsole is no longer providing cushioning or support. Remember that the cushioning effect of the shoe wears out before it looks worn out. If you set your shoes on a level surface, and they tilt in or out, they have begun to break down and will no longer support you. Nagging foot, knee, back, or hip pain may be another signal that you need new footwear.

Good shoes help maintain balance and leg alignment when walking or running. If you have knee problems caused by flat feet or overpronated feet (that roll inward), or a very high-arched foot, then you may need to select running or walking shoes specifically designed for your foot type. If you cannot find comfort and support in standard shoe wear, you may need orthotics. These should be fitted by a professional. After you get orthotics, you may need to change your running shoes to optimize the fit.

7. **Correct Your Gait**

   When your knees hurt, you may unconsciously
   change the way you walk to compensate for the
   pain. If your gait has changed, talk with your
   doctor or physical therapist to see what you need
   to do to correct this. The temporary use of a knee
   support or a more complex orthopedic brace
   may be useful to stabilize your knee and normalize
   your gait.

8. **Seek Softer Ground**

   If you normally walk or exercise along cement
   sidewalks, try walking in the park instead. A simple
   switch to grass can dramatically cut the impact and
   strain you put on your knees. Walking on the firm
   sand on a beach is also a way to ease the impact on
   your knees if you are lucky enough to have access
   to the seashore, while walking or running on soft
   sand will be much more challenging.

9. **Get a Third Leg**

   A cane can help take weight off a painful knee by
   allowing you to lean on it for support and ease
   some weight off your knees. It can also help you
   achieve better balance. Your physical therapist can
   show you how to utilize your cane. If you feel
   self-conscious walking with a cane, invest in an
   attractive or unusual cane.

10. **Get Out of Bed Correctly**

    Get in and out of bed carefully if you have knee
    pain or injury. Roll onto your side and your elbow

and push yourself up with your lower arm while sliding your legs off the edge of the bed. The weight of your legs will swing your chest up with the support of your arm against the bed. Do the reverse to get back into bed. Shift your upper body weight to the palm of your hand resting on the bed. Lower your body slowly, shifting your weight to your forearm, elbow, and shoulder while you swing your legs up to the bed. Try to keep your back straight.

If you have arthritis or stiff knees, doing some simple range-of-motion exercises before getting out of bed can help a lot!

11. **Make Your Home Knee Friendly**
More accidents happen in the home than anywhere else. People bump into poorly placed furniture, they trip over loose scatter rugs or a doorjamb, get caught in a stray wire, and so on. Banging your already sensitive knees on a sharp edge of a low table will cause pain and swelling. Go through your home and assess what is unsafe. For example, do you have sturdy handrails on all stairways? Are your rugs kept in place with slipproof rug pads? Is there a loose wire you will trip over? Do you aggravate your knee pain by kneeling to get things from low cabinets?

12. **Be Smart about Exercise**
If you have chronic knee pain, you may need to change the way you exercise. Don't stop being active, but be smart about when and how you

work out. If your knees ache after jogging or playing basketball—sports that give your knees a pounding—consider switching to swimming, water aerobics, or other low-impact activities at least a few days a week. Sometimes, just limiting or modifying high-impact activities will provide relief.

13. **Warm Up First and Cool Down Last**
Warm up before any physical activity so that little by little the heart rate increases and muscle blood flow improves. Always warm up and stretch and cool down before and after physical activity.

14. **Don't Be a Weekend Warrior**
Someone who exercises on a regular basis is less likely to be injured than someone who does it only on weekends with high intensity. A competitive tennis game on the weekend after spending your week at a desk may predispose you to injury. If you haven't exercised in a while because of travel, work, or illness, start up again slowly. Never try to make up for a lost week of running by doubling your mileage the next week.

15. **Take a Day Off**
If you run or play sports every day of the week, take a day off to rest your body and your knees. Also, if you are an athlete in training, take a light training week every four to six weeks. An alternative to this is cross training, where you

change the type of exercise to provide relative rest to different parts of your body.

16. **Utilize Your Pain Medication Effectively**

Think ahead about demands on your knees. If you know that walking causes pain in your knees, and you want to visit a museum, consider using acetaminophen or an NSAID forty-five minutes before you begin the activity. Take extra care to follow the dosing schedules of prescription or over-the-counter medication. If you are using over-the-counter medication on a regular basis, discuss this with your physician to make sure that you are using these medications in a safe manner.

17. **Gradual Is Good**

Don't increase mileage or intensity too quickly whether you are running, swimming, cycling, or skiing. This is the number one mistake that people make that can predispose to overuse injury. If you are currently running twenty miles a week, increase your total weekly mileage by no more than two to four miles the next week. A periodic long run is part of race preparation, but you should reduce other training components or introduce a day of rest. Change only one training component (distance, time, or speed) at a time.

18. **Avoid Jet Lag in the Knees**

Being jammed into a coach seat on a long flight can leave anyone with sore and stiff knees by the time she reaches her destination. If you have knee problems, try to get a seat where you have more leg room. Flex and extend your knees, try some seated leg raises, and take a walk through the cabin. If you get off the plane, and your knees hurt, rest and stretch. Try to avoid alcohol and coffee on the flight. These can exacerbate jet lag, which, in turn, could further impair your sleep, increase muscle tension, make your pain worse, and interfere with normal daytime activity.

19. Listen to Your Body

Never ignore the warning signs of an injury. Don't continue to train with pain. This is a sure way to prolong your recovery. If your knees hurt, or you are tired, take a break. You are more likely to hurt yourself when you are fatigued. If rest does not resolve your symptoms, see a doctor.

20. Avoid the Last Run

If you are a skier, avoid the tendency to do the last run when you are tired, cold, or fatigued. But it doesn't only apply to skiing. If you are playing tennis, swimming laps, running, or doing any activity, and you are fatigued, unsteady, or stiff and sore, this is a signal from your body to stop.

GLOSSARY

aerobic exercise: activity that benefits the cardiovascular system, such as running.

allograft: a graft from a tissue bank used to reconstruct a ligament, for example.

anaerobic exercise: means "without air"—short, rapid burst of energy such as weight lifting or sprinting.

anterior cruciate ligament: crisscrosses in front of the knee; most frequently injured of the four knee ligaments.

anterior knee pain syndrome: chronic pain in front of the knee.

apophysis: See *growth plate*.

arthrocentesis: draining fluid from the knee joint.

arthroscope: fiber-optic endoscope used inside a joint for surgery or diagnosis.

arthroscopy: surgery using arthroscopic techniques.

articular cartilage: smooth, shiny material that covers bone surfaces where they touch so they can glide easily.

autograft: a piece of tissue taken from your own body to use in another part of your body, such as in ligament reconstruction.

autologous chondrocyte implantation: a technique of harvesting healthy cartilage cells, cultivating them in a lab, and then implanting them at the site of cartilage loss.

avascular necrosis: the death of bone tissue caused by lack of blood supply.

biofeedback: a technique of training yourself with electronic devices to modify autonomic body functions such as the perception of pain.

biologic response modifiers: a new class of genetically engineered drugs that block the immune system from causing inflammation (see *disease modifying antirheumatic drugs*).

Blount's disease: a condition affecting children that causes the legs to bow.

bursa: a fluid-filled sac formed by two layers of synovial tissue that facilitates gliding; many are strategically located around joints (plural is *bursae*).

bursitis: inflammation of a bursa.

calcium pyrophosphate: body chemical that can cause pseudogout, a painful inflammatory condition.

chondroitin sulfate: nutritional supplement, a component of normal cartilage often used in combination with glucosamine to relieve arthritis pain.

chondromalacia of the patella: pain caused by damage to the cartilage lining of the patella.

corticosteroids: man-made drugs similar to the hormone cortisol produced by the adrenal glands and used to relieve joint inflammation and pain.

debridement: an arthroscopic technique for "flushing out" loose particles of cartilage from the knee joint.

discoid meniscus: abnormal meniscus that is round rather than *C*-shaped.

disease modifying antirheumatic drugs (DMARDs): drugs that slow down or prevent the immune system from attacking the knees, which in turn prevents swelling and pain.

distal: farthest away from the point of connection.

femur: thigh bone.

fibrocartilage: cartilage that contains collagen fibers and is more elastic than articular cartilage. The meniscus is made of fibrocartilage.

fibula: a long, narrow bone in the shin alongside the larger tibia.

Gerdy's tubercle: the attachment site of the iliotibial band to the tibia.

glucosamine: a nutritional supplement made from shells of crab, lobster, and shrimp, and marketed as a pain reducer for mild arthritis.

gluteal muscles: buttocks muscles.

gout: a form of arthritis that affects men more than women.

growth plate: an area of specialized cartilage present near the end of long bones (also called the physis), where longitudinal growth of bone occurs until skeletal maturity.

hamstring muscles: the long muscles in the back of the thighs.

hip abductor muscles: muscles from the hip down the thigh to help rotate the thigh.

hyaluronic acid: See *viscosupplementation*.

hyperuricemia: buildup of uric acid in the blood; a condition related to gout.

iliotibial band (ITB): a long, fibrous structure extending from the outside top of the femur to the outside top of the tibia.

iliotibial band syndrome: a chronic, painful condition of the ITB caused by overuse.

intravenous (IV): method of injecting or infusing medications directly into the bloodstream.

jumper's knee: an overuse injury, patellar tendinitis.

juvenile rheumatoid arthritis (JRA): an autoimmune system disorder that attacks the synovial tissue of the joints; the only type of arthritis to affect children.

knock-kneed: malformation of the legs that cause the knees to be too close together.

lateral collateral ligament: ligament that supports the outer aspect of the knee.

lateral release: a surgical procedure to cut a tight ligament to allow the patella to resume a normal position.

ligaments: fibrous bands of tissue that support the knee.

maltracking: a condition where the patella moves abnormally toward the outside of the knee in the trochlear groove.

medial collateral ligament: the ligament at the inner side of the knee.

medial patellofemoral ligament (MPFL): a supporting structure important to patella stability.

meniscectomy: surgery to repair a torn piece of meniscus.

menisci: plural for meniscus; each knee has two menisci.

meniscus: *C*-shaped pad of cartilage that separates the surfaces of the femur and tibia.

mosaicplasty: known as osteochondral grafting, a technique to replace lost cartilage and bone with new plugs of cartilage and bone taken from another area.

nonsteroidal anti-inflammatory drugs (NSAIDs): drugs such as aspirin that relieve inflammation.

open reduction internal fixation (ORIF): surgery that uses screws, plates, and/or rods to repair fractures.

orthotic device: a wedge or platform used in a shoe to correct an imbalance in leg length or position.

Osgood-Schlatter disease: an overuse condition that causes knee pain at the attachment of the patellar tendon to the tibia in children and adolescents who are still growing.

osteoarthritis: a condition caused by degeneration of the articular cartilage that leads to chronic inflammation and pain.

osteochondral fracture: a bone fracture that also damages the articular cartilage.

osteochondritis dissecans (OCD): a condition where blood is not getting to an area of cartilage and bone, causing them to become separated from their original positions.

osteotomy: surgery to realign the knee joint and relieve pressure on the side damaged from osteoarthritis; an alternative to knee replacement.

patella: kneecap, a small, triangular bone in front of the knee.

patellar dislocation: a kneecap that has dislodged from the trochlear groove.

patellar subluxation: a kneecap that is transiently not tracking correctly in the trochlear groove.

patellofemoral joint: where the end of the femur meets the patella, in the trochlear groove.

patellofemoral pain: pain in and around the kneecap.

physis: See *growth plate.*

pigmented villonodular synovitis (PVNS): benign tumor of the synovial tissue.

posterior cruciate ligament: one of two ligaments that connects the femur and tibia.

prosthesis: an artificial replacement for a body part, such as a knee.

proximal: closest to the point of connection.

pseudogout: a condition similar to gout, but caused by an excess of pyrophosphate calcium crystals rather than uric acid crystals.

psoriatic arthritis: arthritis that may develop in someone who has the skin condition psoriasis.

purines: natural substances in the body's cells and in foods, but certain foods such as organ meats have high concentrations.

retinaculum: a band of fibrous tissue that helps support the patella.

rheumatoid arthritis: an autoimmune disease that attacks the articular cartilage in joints.

runner's knee: patellofemoral pain in front of the knee.

septic arthritis: arthritis that is caused by a joint infection.

subluxation: a condition where the kneecap is not situated properly (loose or tilted) within the trochlear groove.

synovial fluid: See *synovium*.

synovium: thin membrane that lines the knee joint and creates synovial fluid, a lubricant for the joint.

tendinitis: inflammation of a tendon.

tendinosis: an acute and chronic degeneration of the tendons caused by trauma or age.

tendons: tough, fibrous bands of tissue, the strongest in the body, which connect muscles to bone.

tibia: the long calf bone that connects to the knee.

tibial tubercle: where the patellar tendon attaches to the tibia.

transcutaneous electrical nerve stimulation (TENS): the use of electrical stimulation to diminish the body's processing of pain impulses.

trochlear groove: an indentation (like a track) at the end of the femur, in which the patella glides so the knee can bend and straighten.

viscosupplementation: injection of synthetic fluids that mimic synovial fluid, such as hyaluronic acid, into the knee joint to relieve pain.

APPENDIX

INFORMATION RESOURCES

American Academy of Orthopaedic Surgeons
PO Box 1998
Des Plaines, IL 60017-1998
Phone: 847-823-7186 or 800-824-BONE
www.aaos.org

The Academy provides education and practice management services for orthopedic surgeons and allied health professionals and patients. It also serves as an advocate for improved patient care and informs the public about the science of orthopedics. The orthopedist's scope of practice includes disorders of the body's bones, joints, ligaments, muscles, and tendons. The Academy produces a variety of educational programs and information brochures that are free to the public. For a single copy of an AAOS brochure, send a self-addressed stamped envelope to the address above, or visit the website.

American Medical Association
515 North State Street
Chicago, IL 60610
800-621-8335
www.ama-assn.org

Click on "Find a Doctor."

American Orthopaedic Society for Sports Medicine
6300 N. River Road, Suite 500
Rosemont, IL 60018
847-292-4900
Fax: 847-292-4905
www.sportsmed.org
General information: aossm@aossm.org

This is a professional organization for physicians. In addition to a directory of members, it will help you find a doctor. Patient information about common sports-related orthopedic conditions is also available on this site.

American Physical Therapy Association
1111 North Fairfax Street
Alexandria, VA 22314
Phone: 703-684-2782 or 800-999-APTA
www.apta.org

The goal of the American Physical Therapy Association is to foster advancements in physical therapy practice, research, and education. The Association publishes a free brochure titled "Taking Care of the Knees."

Arthritis Foundation
PO Box 7669
Atlanta, GA 30357-0669
Phone: 404-872-7100 or 800-568-4045
www.arthritis.org

The Foundation has several free brochures about the various forms of arthritis that affect the knee, coping with arthritis, arthritis treatment, and exercise. A free brochure on protecting your joints is titled "Using Your Joints

Wisely." The Foundation can also provide addresses and phone numbers for local chapters and physician and clinic referrals.

CastleConnolly.com
"Find a Doctor" link. Physician profiles are selected after peer nomination, extensive research, and careful review and screening by its own physician-directed research team.

Hospital for Special Surgery
535 East 70th Street
New York, NY 10021
Phone: 212-224-7900
www.hss.edu

The Hospital for Special Surgery is ranked number one in the United States for orthopedics by *U.S. News & World Report,* and third for rheumatology. Physicians and scientists at HSS pioneered the first total knee replacement and have perfected surgical techniques for minimally invasive hip and knee replacement surgery. HSS has the largest sports medicine faculty in the country and the first Women's Sports Medicine Center.

National Institute of Arthritis and Musculoskeletal and Skin Diseases
National Institutes of Health
1 AMS Circle
Bethesda, MD 20892
Phone: 301-495-4484 or 877-22-NIAMS
TTY: 301-565-2966

NIAMSInfo@mail.nih.gov

www.niams.nih.gov

NIAMS provides information about various forms of arthritis and rheumatic diseases as well as other bone, muscle, joint, and skin diseases. It distributes educational information for patients and refers people to other sources of information.

INDEX

Page numbers in *italics* refer to illustrations.